M000313314

HUMAN
WELL-BEING
IN THE LIGHT OF
EVOLUTION

KEVIN HOLBROOK

Copyright © 2014 Kevin Holbrook

All rights reserved.

A Pinion Press First Print Edition

PINION
press

ISBN-13: 978-0692229323 (Pinion Press)

ISBN-10: 0692229329

Cover by Kevin Holbrook

Disclaimer: The ideas, concepts, and opinions contained herein are not intended to be personal, medical, or health advice. This book is sold with the understanding that author and publisher are not offering medical advice of any kind. Always consult and receive clearance from a licensed health professional before changing lifestyle habits. By reading this book you acknowledge that your health and happiness are your own responsibility — not the author's/publisher's.

Author and publisher claim no responsibility to any person or entity for any liability, loss, or damage caused or alleged to be caused directly or indirectly as a result of the use, application or interpretation of the material in this book.

The Food and Drug Administration has not evaluated the statements contained herein.

"Nothing in biology makes sense
except in the light of evolution."

Theodosius Dobzhansky PhD

geneticist and evolutionary biologist

"Nothing in medicine makes sense
except in the light of evolution."

Randolph Nesse MD

physician and evolutionary biologist

George C. Williams PhD

evolutionary biologist

Ajit Varki PhD

physician-scientist, cellular and molecular medicine

"Nothing in popular culture makes sense
except in the light of evolution."

Gad Saad PhD

behavioral scientist

"Nothing in morality makes sense
except in the light of evolution."

Joshua Tybur PhD

social psychologist

"Nothing in psychology makes sense
except in the light of evolution."

Joel Guarna PhD

clinical psychologist

Para Mamá.

Todo lo que tengo, tú me lo has dado.

CONTENTS

"Evolution is a light which illuminates all facts,
a curve that all lines must follow."

Pierre Teilhard de Chardin

Jesuit priest

PREFACE

To many, it's a dangerous idea. It threatens to replace old beliefs, to change the world we built and the values we guard, even those deemed sacred. It's an ugly idea that has been taken too far before, one besmirched by elders and stained by the course of history.

It's the idea that we are animals; that we evolved here on the earth of Earth like primates; that we came down from the trees, used tools, walked upright, controlled fire, developed language, became intelligent, and started farming; that we built this crazy civilization with nothing but our free hands and big brains. It's the idea that civilization is not the place our bodies, hearts, and minds belong. It's the idea that we can do better.

I wrote this book because it's the book I always wanted to read but no one had written. It's a book that will explore evolution and human well-being in the most important ways: revealing the truth about the human animal inside all of us, and what that means for our day-to-day lives.

In the chapters that follow, I play the role of journalist, researcher, and interpreter. I did the hard work of digging through academic journals, learning the nuances of evolutionary theory, perusing the work of scientists and thought leaders, building on their ideas, exploring strategies, and then presenting it all in a clear, concise, comprehensive format.

This book will ask you to open your mind, to sharpen your critical thinking methodology, and to heighten your standards of evidence. This book is an exercise in logic and strategy, driven by science and research. My goal is that you'll see yourself in a new light, and come out the other end a better person for it. And in the end, you may find that what defines our species is the very thing that makes us human.

Viva la evolución.

"To be godly yet creaturely is impossibly cruel."

Jason Silva

futurist and filmmaker

INTRODUCTION

The premise of this book is that you are an evolved organism, a collection of compromising evolved traits that were subject to the ancestral environment over the course of millions of years of evolution extending all the way back to the first lifeform on Earth. Have you ever considered what this means for your day-to-day life?

The truth of evolution has broad, profound applications to nearly all areas of life. You can measure the magnitude of evolution's promise by the breadth of its academic disciplines, a plethoric list long enough to fill this page. Evolution is the unifying theory of the life sciences, the guiding principle of biology. It is the only intellectually satisfying source for answers about human behavior, human biology, human origins, and human relationships — questions that matter to us all. In truth, only evolution intellectually satisfies life's biggest questions. Who are we? Where do we come from? What does it mean to be human?

So why not ask questions of evolution about our everyday lives as well? Can we stand to gain from an evolutionary perspective on the natural human diet? Will our exercise routine become smarter by understanding musculoskeletal adaptation, natural human locomotion, and genetic expression? Shall we sleep better if we understand and leverage the adaptive traits that govern our sleep cycles? Can we win respect and friendship by understanding the dynamics of social status, bonding, and human interaction? And what about lofty abstractions like love, happiness, and virtue? Are these not simply traits subject to our evolved psychology? Are they not more attainable once understood?

Starting this book, I was shocked that so many before me had not asked these fundamental questions. I grew up in the intellectual climate of Silicon Valley and the San Francisco Bay Area, and I have long been familiar with the truth of evolution. But it was the *interpretation* of human evolution that fascinated me. If we are animals, then what does that mean for our lives?

This is a topic that has become increasingly important over the last decade with popular evolutionists and small, thriving countercultures. Gyms like Crossfit, which incorporate natural movement, now seem to pop up in cities across America and the world; barefoot running is enjoying a resurgence; and diets based wholly or partly on evolution — the Paleo Diet, the Caveman Diet, the Real Food Diet, the Zone Diet, the Low Carb Diet , the Weston A. Price Diet, the Primal Blueprint, the Ketogenic Diet, the Evolution Diet, Protein Power, the Stone Age Diet, the Bond Effect, the Warrior Diet, the Raw Diet, and others — have helped countless people reverse disease, improve health, lead more fulfilling lives, and, yes, finally get their six-pack abs. It's a revolutionary idea that acknowledges a simple truth. That you are an animal.

This book aims to take that truth to the most important places. It's going to look at major topics in physical and mental health in order to see them more clearly, but it will also present reasonable and actionable strategies based on the evolutionary interpretation of each topic. Many of the conclusions to follow will legitimate some conventional wisdoms, overturn others, and ultimately take us to a new understanding of what it means to be healthy, happy, and human.

And so I'll ask you: are you healthy? I mean, are you *really* healthy? It's a legitimate question, because most people think they are — when in reality they are not.[1] And like almost everything, evolution explains this.

It's called the 'optimism bias': the human penchant to think things are better than they really are. It's one more fascinating example of the work of evolution. An installation in the *Handbook of Evolutionary Psychology* states,

> ...trying and failing may not matter very much, whereas failing
> to try could be very costly, at least relative to competitors. Thus,

---

[1] Weinstein (1980). Unrealistic optimism about future life events. *Journal of Personal and Social Psychology* 39: 806-820.

evolution can be expected to produce mechanisms biased toward positive illusion...[2]

Evolution has given us the gift and curse of optimism that you see every day. You see it in chain smokers who think *their* odds for disease are lower than the *actual odds for disease.* You see it in motorcyclists who think they can beat the odds of a crash. And you see it in normal folks who think they are doing just fine.

But normal folks are not doing just fine. Half of all Americans are on prescription drugs.[3] The majority of us are overweight or obese. According to American Psychiatric Association standards, about half of us will develop a mental illness in our lives.[4] *Time* magazine reports, "we spend more on healthcare than the next 10 biggest spenders combined: Japan, Germany, France, China, the U.K., Italy, Canada, Brazil, Spain and Australia."[5] We have more sick people *and* more expensive care. America, the most industrialized country in the world, predictably leads the pack in sickness, but this isn't just about America. This is about all civilized, industrialized societies.

Normal everyday people who think themselves healthy see all kinds of adverse symptoms, many of which are considered a normal part of life. They have trouble sleeping. Their energy levels swing wildly. They have asthma, acne, headaches, back pain, dry skin, chapped lips, crooked teeth, rotting gums, itchy eyes, acid reflux, stomach aches, overactive sweat glands, constant allergies — and *yet they are healthy?* And this is just part of the picture. Add 'normal' mental afflictions like anxiety, chronic stress, low self-esteem, loneliness, and sadness, and you've got a world of people living in delusion.

These are just some among many of the diseases of civilization that

---

[2] Haselton, Nettle, and Andrews. "The Evolution of Cognitive Bias." *Handbook of Evolutionary Psychology.* [Ed. David Buss]. Wiley, 2005. pp. 738-39.

[3] National Center for Health Statistics. "NCHS Data Brief No. 42, September 2010."

[4] Kessler et al (2005). Lifetime prevalence and age-of-onset distributions of DSM-IV disorders in the National Comorbidity Survey Replication. *Arch. Gen. Psychiatry* 62 (6): 593–602.

[5] Brill, Steven. "Bitter Pill: Why Medical Bills are Killing Us." *Time Magazine.* Retrieved from http://healthland.time.com/2013/02/20/bitter-pill-why-medical-bills-are-killing-us/2/

ravage the human population. The big killers are heart disease, cancer, obesity, and stroke. Many people consider them normal because they happen often, not realizing that 'normal' in the context of civilization isn't normal at all, because evolution teaches us one more burning truth — that the human species is resilient.

We are the products of billions of years of evolution. Have you ever considered what that means? The implications are staggering. *We are the descendants of winners undefeated in a billion-year game to stay alive.* Every ancestor before you — every generation of ancestors — was strong enough to survive and reproduce. Think about it. Where other organisms have failed, humans are here today precisely *because* we are hard to kill. It's a shocking statistic: 99% of all life that has ever lived on Earth is now extinct. We are the 1%. Do you think humanity thrives on Earth because we are sick and fragile, sad and dumb?

There is only one good explanation for the prevalence of disease and personal anguish in contemporary society, and it has everything to do with evolution. Our evolving minds and bodies do not fit the sick structure of society. We are bombarded with things that are unnatural in evolutionary terms: toxins, pathogens, chronic stress, and social disconnection— things that were introduced recently with civilization. Our lives are almost completely out of line with the environment that shaped our minds and bodies. Understanding evolution can help us solve this problem, not by going back but by adapting forward.

Evolutionists know that genes aren't there to cause disease,[6] that food isn't there to make us fat, that air isn't there to give us asthma, that the sun isn't there to give us cancer, that our bodies *want* to move playfully, that sadness isn't there to make us clinically depressed, that our species is optimistic and joyful naturally, that empathy should be ubiquitous, that egalitarianism is in our nature, that overwhelming love and happiness are real, even if they are hard to achieve, even if the structure of society is vying against us at every turn. We got lost somewhere along the way and the reason why

---

[6] A refrain in Matt Ridley's *Genome*, which he writes in all caps repeatedly.

may be hard to swallow.

You've been lied to.

You've been lied to by nearly everyone.

You've been lied to by the people you trust. Nutritionists who told you to drink processed skim milk for bone health and to cook with vegetable oils that aren't even made from vegetables. Journalists who misinterpret study findings or sensationalize them, often regurgitating the status quo. News outlets that pick stories in order to attract eyeballs for advertisements. (I would know. I worked in news advertising.) Doctors who promise to heal you by prescribing drugs to abate symptoms — drugs that *don't even address the root cause* of those symptoms.

You've been lied to by the people you empower. Health officials who mandate the alarming standards for school lunches. Governments who protect big farm subsidies or even insist that we need them. Representatives that have to balance your voting interest against the financial interests that keep them in power and fuel their careers. Regulators who allow outlandish health claims on food labels, like "heart-healthy" sugar-coated breakfast cereals.

You've been lied to by the people you support. Gyms lined with treadmills promising to melt the fat away. Early-morning boot camps that plan to get you fit by beating the hell out of your sleep-deprived body. Gimmicky products that are supposed to make you beautiful but are only a pathological attempt to take your money.

And you've been lied to by yourself. Blinded by limited perspective and fed conflicting information, we struggle to find the truth. We hold on to our cozy delusions and the conventions of old. We find comfort in the lies, often unable to accept ideas unless they jive with all the other preconceived notions already floating in our heads, the flotsam of human experience. An idea overheard on the radio or advice casually shared at a party — there is no backbone to the things that guide most decisions.

Only evolution reveals the depth of sadness in a tribeless human, disconnected from the nurture of mother Earth, sickened by the structure of society, taught to replace the boundless love of clan with the simplicity of the nuclear family, left often with shallow friendships unfit for the most highly evolved of social brains and emotional hearts, indoctrinated against the instinct of egalitarianism, enslaved by socio-economic class and corporate hierarchy, kept from the blanket of freedom in which every wild soul is born.

Evolution is revelatory. After years of study, I now look at a world mired in fallacy, largely based on norms. People follow the pack, latch onto the latest trends, and they do so as naturally as a flock of birds changing direction in flight. Animals do this naturally; they conform to the behavior of others within their group because it's safer than deviation. Game theorists have proven this true, and only evolution explains this fascinating topic that we will explore later. I see people taking measured steps toward their goals based on these social mores. But this is a problem, because in today's world "normal" is benign at best, detrimental at worst, and suboptimal for certain. To address this problem, we have to start with the way that we think.

We need to learn how to think about human well-being. We need to step back and embed our knowledge within a logical framework. We need to ask the big questions. We need to uncover what's true, even the hard truths, the dark truths, perhaps those are the most important of all. We need to erect the walls of logic in this maze, solidify them with the strength of science, and explore them with the map of strategy.

Well, that's what you're holding in your hands. Three hundred academic references in as many pages of blood, sweat, and tears. I mean that quite literally. I rolled the dice on three years of my life, a personal sacrifice for doing what I see as some of the most important work of our time.

This book is a comprehensive look at human well-being in the light of evolution. Welcome to the rabbit hole, because this book is the red pill, and you're about to swallow it.

INTRODUCTION

"A scientific truth does not triumph by convincing its opponents and making them see the light, but rather because its opponents eventually die and a new generation grows up that is familiar with it."

Max Planck

discoverer of quantum physics

CHAPTER 1

FOUNDATIONS FOR DECISION-MAKING: SCIENCE, LOGIC, AND STRATEGY

Science is a process for building and organizing knowledge in the form of testable theories, facts, and predictions about the natural world. Classically, science refers to the body of knowledge itself, of the type that can be rationally or logically explained.[7] But in today's most strict terms, science is a lengthy experimental process characterized by control, precision, skepticism, discourse, and repeatability.[8] The goal of science is to know and understand the nature of the world *according to the highest standards of evidence*. It is the objective quest for truth.

For example, gravity. Say you notice that things fall, so you form a hypothesis: there's a law of nature called gravity that makes things fall. (Excuse my oversimplification here, for the sake of argument.) To prove this scientifically, you conduct a series of experiments. You control every variable of the experiment: what is falling, how it is falling, everything. You take specific measurements. You conduct experiments until you have enough data.

---

[7] J. L. Heilbron, ed. *The Oxford Companion to the History of Modern Science*. New York: Oxford University Press, 2003.

[8] Gauch Jr., Hugh G. *Scientific Method in Practice*. New York: Cambridge University Press, 2003.

After experimentation, you find that you were right: things did fall according to your gravity idea. You publish your findings in a respected peer-reviewed academic journal. *It isn't until now that your hypothesis is a full-fledged theory.*

You'll have a slow, healthy discourse with other scientists around the world who nitpick the meaning and complexity of your theory for a long, long time while other similar experiments are done and published and talked about. The theory itself may evolve as new knowledge refines or corrects the precise definition of gravity. Scientists will slowly accept this theory, then all of them will, and then they will build upon your gravity theory with other interconnected theories. It has taken a long time, but it isn't until now that, finally, your gravity theory is considered true and can then comfortably and casually be referred to as fact. In this way, gravity is still a theory, but it is also considered a scientific fact, as it should be, because the overwhelming evidence leads to that conclusion. It would be unreasonable — indeed, even perverse — to reject a theory so often confirmed and validated over time.

I mean only to highlight the degree to which evolution is true, because evolution is a scientific fact.[9] [10] It has gone through all of the stages of the scientific process. It is universally accepted among scientists from a spectrum of disciplines. There are layers of evolutionary theory, and evolution is reaffirmed over and over again in observation and experimentation. Yesterday, today, and tomorrow, a scientist somewhere will discover or explore something related to evolution that will further confirm, build upon, or refine what we already know a great deal about. Humans have recreated some of the processes of evolution via artificial selection (like in dog breeding) and have observed and documented speciation (the introduction of new species), both of which are predictable within evolutionary theory. Thanks to new fields like genetics and epigenetics, we now know more about evolution than Darwin ever thought possible.

Evolution is the unifying theory of the life sciences. It is the most

---

[9] National Academy of Science Institute of Medicine. *Science, Evolution, and Creationism*. National Academy Press, 2008.

[10] Coyne, Jerry. *Why Evolution is True*. New York: Penguin, 2009.

important idea in all of biology, arguably the most important idea that has occurred to anyone in the history of human thought. It is totally, universally, incontrovertibly true according to the highest standards of evidence that human beings have ever devised. Theodosius Dobzhansky, the prominent geneticist and evolutionary biologist, once said, "Nothing in biology makes sense except in the light of evolution." Indeed, nothing in life makes sense except in the light of evolution. This is true for all of the topics in this book, as you will see.

Evolution: Fact or Theory?

There is some difference in the scientific community over the language of science in regard to what exactly constitute facts, laws, theories, axioms, etc. Some people retain strict semantics, arguing that all scientific theories are eternal — that theories never fall into the realm of 'fact'. Facts, they argue, are what theories are based on. As an alternative, they refer to proven theories as being 'true'. This is contrary to the common understanding of fact, which is simply defined as an idea that is true. In this way, evolution is both a theory and a fact, depending on who you are talking to.

However, this debate is largely irrelevant to our purposes because it merely nitpicks at linguistic lines. It does not change the validity of the evolutionary model, which is itself universally regarded as scientifically sound. I personally refer to evolution as fact — as I do gravity — because it would be ridiculous not to consider it one. (I also commonly use the phrase 'evolutionary theory', not to discount its truth, but to highlight the diverse intersectional ideas within it.) In this way, evolution becomes the 'fact' for further theories. It is the foundation upon which we build more advanced knowledge; it is the stable ground for the arguments, assertions, inferences, and premises in the coming chapters.

The Drawbacks of Science

"Don't trust anyone over thirty."

Jack Weinberg, American activist

While science can herald certain theories and bring them into the light of truth, there are arenas where general scientific endeavor leaves us lacking. This may be due to the abstract nature of the field (sociology), the complex nature of the field (psychology), or the physical limitations of evidence (history/archeology). Despite the fact that the arduous standards of science are useful in nearly every realm of human knowledge, sometimes science is simply not enough to reach a conclusion on a given topic in our time. For many subjects, it will take decades more to answer today's questions. And the more we understand, the more new questions are born.

Science can also be untrustworthy, even in the venerable field of medicine. In the words of Marcia Angell, former editor of the *New England Journal of Medicine*, arguably the most respected medical journal in the world,

> It is simply no longer possible to believe much of the clinical research that is published, or to rely on the judgment of trusted physicians or authoritative medical guidelines. I take no pleasure in this conclusion, which I reached slowly and reluctantly over my two decades as an editor of *The New England Journal of Medicine.*[11]

Here, Angell is addressing the interplay between drug company clinical trials and their effect on doctor recommendations. It should go without saying that drug companies and the medical field can save lives, mitigate terrible

---

[11] Angell, Marcia (2009). Drug Companies & Doctors: a Story of Corruption. *New York Review of Books* [Web file]. Retrieved from http://www.nybooks.com/articles/archives/2009/jan/15/drug-companies-doctorsa-story-of-corruption/?pagination=false

symptoms, and advance human health in myriad ways — a fact that history teaches us well. Indeed, drug companies and medical institutions play an important role in human progress. Instead, Angell's statement highlights simply that science is subject to forces that weaken it. We must acknowledge these forces if we're ever to improve upon them.

Medical science has received its fair share of criticism from within the medical community itself. John Ioannidis is a professor and chairman at Tufts University School of Medicine. His 2005 paper about the drawbacks of science was the most downloaded item of the academic journal *PLOS Medicine*. The paper, provocatively titled, "Why Most Published Research Findings Are False," states,

> Simulations show that for most study designs and settings, it is more likely for a research claim to be false than true. Moreover, for many current scientific fields, claimed research findings may often be simply accurate measures of the prevailing bias.[12]

Ioannidis covers many factors that may contribute to false conclusions:

> In this framework, a research finding is less likely to be true when the studies conducted in a field are smaller; when effect sizes are smaller; when there is a greater number and lesser preselection of tested relationships; where there is greater flexibility in designs, definitions, outcomes, and analytical modes; when there is greater financial and other interest and prejudice; and when more teams are involved in a scientific field in chase of statistical significance.

Ioannidis had analyzed "49 of the most important research findings over the

---

[12] Ioannidis JPA (2005) Why Most Published Research Findings Are False. *PLoS Medicine* 2(8): e124.

last 13 years" and "45 claimed to have uncovered effective interventions. Thirty-four of these claims had been retested, and 14 of these, or 41 percent, had been convincingly shown to be wrong or significantly exaggerated."[13] [14] That's almost half of critically important medical claims. Disturbing, to say the least. Many people rely on doctors for relief from suffering and place great trust in them in times of need.

Medicine also severely lacks the incorporation of evolutionary theory. A 2012 paper aptly titled, "Nothing in Medicine Makes Sense Except in the Light of Evolution," states,

> The near complete absence of evolution in medical school curricula is a historical anomaly that needs correction. Otherwise, we will continue to train generations of physicians who lack understanding of some fundamental principles that should guide both medical practice and research.[15]

The common understanding of medicine must acknowledge its strengths and weaknesses in order to understand it for what it is, and perhaps to change it for the better.

Science also often sees conflicts of interest, misinterpretations by the media, or deliberate fraud by the scientists themselves. Many studies are bankrolled by the organizations that stand to gain from the science being done, which, in turn, places pressure on the findings and the careers of scientists conducting the study. A recent review found that studies with financial conflicts of interests are five times more likely to find no link

---

[13] Freedman, D (2010). "Lies, Damned Lies, and Medical Science". *The Atlantic* [Web file] Retrieved from http://www.theatlantic.com/magazine/print/2010/11/lies-damned-lies-and-medical-science/308269/

[14] Ioannidis, J (2005). Contradicted and initially stronger effects in highly cited clinical research. *Journal of the American Medical Association* 294(2):218-28.

[15] Varki, A (2012). Nothing in medicine makes sense except in the light of evolution. *Journal of Molecular Medicine* 90 (5): 481-494.

between sugar-sweetened beverages and weight gain.[16] It should be no mystery why this is the case once you follow the money and identify the incentives guiding the behavior of those involved.

Journalists reporting on a complex study may exaggerate, distort, or 'spin' the facts, intentionally or unintentionally, according to their own biases, ignorance, and/or career pressure. Look how desperately news teams emphasize stories that are dramatic, shocking, and engaging. This is simply capitalism, a quest to boost viewership/readership, in order to rake in more advertising dollars. Most of these are private, profit-seeking corporations, after all. They're not evil, it's just business.

And lastly, scientists do commit fraud. Scientist Yoshitaka Fujii currently holds the record for the number of fraudulent published scientific papers at 172.[17] This was discovered in 2012. Altogether, these are challenges to human progress, because scientific truths are at the heart of decision-making. Without adequate knowledge and information, we simply can't make the right decisions for ourselves, our community, or our society.

So how can we rectify some of these problems and improve the scientific process?

Darwin's Dictum

"About thirty years ago there was much talk that geologists ought only to observe and not theorize; and I will remember someone saying that at this rate a man might as well go into a gravel-pit and count the pebbles and describe the colours. How odd it is that anyone should not see that all observation must be for or against some view if it is to be of any service!"

Charles Darwin, gentleman scientist

---

[16] Rastrollo et al (2013). Financial conflicts of interest and reporting bias regarding the association between sugar-sweetened beverages and weight gain: a systematic review of systematic reviews. *PLoS Medicine* 10(12): e1001578.

[17] Akst, Jef (2012). "Anesthesiologist Fabricates 172 Papers." *The Scientist.*

Our ideas are stronger when we embed them within a logical framework. Indeed, most sciences do. They uphold a strong central paradigm, worldview, or theoretical model in order to make sense of everything. Physics utilizes quantum theory. Geology leverages the theory of plate tectonics. Chemistry employs atomic theory. And biology applies evolutionary theory. It would seem reasonable, then, that all other biological disciplines, by extension, also incorporate evolutionary theory as a working paradigm. Indeed, most do. Ecology, genetics, anthropology, ethology, zoology, and more, all leverage evolution as a guiding principle. After all, evolution is the unifying theory of the life sciences. If evolution were disproved tomorrow, which is impossible, these disciplines would implode, for the sheer mountain of knowledge they have built on evolutionary theory is too great.

But some disciplines, such as medicine, nutrition, psychology, and public health, do not fully leverage evolutionary theory in their methodology, even despite the fact that biological principles are hugely relevant to their fields. Their worldviews, therefore, can be improved. In fact, many people today are working to do just that. We have seen the rise of Darwinian Medicine, the prolific contributions of Evolutionary Psychology, and the burgeoning field of Ancestral Health — all of which reaffirm the validity of the evolutionary model as a valid paradigm that illuminates the topic of human well-being.

Bad Science: Or, Nutrition Science

One of the important fields science has yet to conquer is nutrition. Information in the nutrition field is highly political, inadequate, and inconsistent. Many studies do not uphold the standards of true science, the results are often misleading or inconsistent, and the conclusions often contradict previous ones.

The track record for nutrition is wholly unimpressive, because it's quite easy to demonstrate how public health has consistently deteriorated over time. Even with sweeping policy changes like low-fat dieting and whole grain recommendations, it's well-known that we are unhealthier than ever. So why would that be? Is it simply the new types of foods available that are increasingly destroying our health, or is something wrong with the system itself?

First, the field of nutrition is heavily influenced by industry and special interest. It's no secret how large companies and collective industries can sway elections, influence policies, or shut out smaller competitors with buyouts or lawsuits. But less commonly known is the degree to which industry influences science.[18] Many published studies are bankrolled by a special interest group, such as the National Dairy Council, a group clearly seeking to increase dairy sales. This conflict of interest is one of the contributing factors to the confusion that surrounds so much of nutrition science. As Upton Sinclair once said, "It's difficult to get a man to understand something when his salary depends on his not understanding it."

Second, the complex realms of science produce endless variables that inevitably alter the results of experimentation, ultimately arising as misleading associations or false conclusions. Due to how studies are conducted, confounding factors can sneak into the data, influencing how variables are correlated. These factors may imply a causal relationship where none exist, because correlation is not causation. Some of the best epidemiological science that we have seeks to control as many variables as possible, but even the best attempts to do so do not uphold the high standards of precision and control that are hallmarks of the scientific process.

Third, much of the experimental nutrition science that exists today is simply inadequate. Experimentation on animals is common, for instance, due to the difficulty of performing long term controlled experiments on humans. But to experiment on a mouse instead of a human is to violate an important control of the experiment: the human. Clearly, mice are not human, therefore the results mean only so much when translating them to the human body or

---

[18] Rowe, Sylvia et al. "Funding food science and nutrition research: financial conflicts and scientific integrity." *The American Journal of Clinical Nutrition.* International Life Sciences Institute, 2009.

mind.

Science is inadequate when the scientific ideals of control, specificity, and repeatability are not met. These are rare in the realm of nutrition science because they are simply not reasonable to pursue. You would have to isolate large groups of people for months or years to control every variable and get 'real science' done. Of course, real science rarely happens. Financing these studies is difficult. Finding participants to meet these demands is nearly impossible. Experimentation to the degree of true scientific rigor rarely happens for these reasons.

This is why health science is dominated by correlative epidemiological studies, many of which are covered by news media. We hear things like, "Milk may increase risk for cancer by 15% percent." How did they get these numbers? They tracked people's habits and health in very unscientific ways, such as surveys and phone calls where people make education guesses about how much milk they drank and report any diseases that arise over time. Then they run the numbers methodically, controlling for certain variables, hoping to find a correlation. If a significant correlation is found, then they have an observation, and the conclusion is limited to: the variables *might* be related. If they don't find a correlation, then they've made a conclusion: the variables are unrelated. It's a common refrain in statistics that *correlation is not causation*, so even if the variables are related, it does not mean that one causes the other. This is captured succinctly in a saying popularized by Mark Twain: "Lies, damned lies, and statistics."

To understand science is to understand that correlative studies like this mean very little. Sure, correlative studies are helpful. Perhaps they are better than nothing. But there are so many conflicting conclusions that come out of these studies, and there are so many confounding variables, that studies like this will be misleading, and therefore potentially deleterious, as often as they will be helpful. The last half century has proven that people should not be getting their information from the news media.

A better route to human knowledge is to move beyond correlations by seeking to *prove* a causal relationship and then working to reveal the biological mechanism in question. That means doing actual studies on humans — randomized double blind controlled trials — and then likely relying on scientific collaboration to demonstrate how the causal relationship actually works in the body. Then, and only then, should we endorse an idea like low-fat dieting. (Our health officials have not done this with low-fat endorsements; they stopped once they had a correlation. In related news, they're dead wrong about fat.) Ultimately, this means raising our standards of evidence.

Should we take correlative studies into consideration? Of course we should. However, correlations, like many of the ones that popularly make the news, are good at best as hypotheses that need to be tested against real science (randomized double blind controlled trials). And as far as hypothesis-building goes, correlations are not all that we have. Fortunately, we have something better than bad science. We have logic.

The Role of Reason

Logic is the study of valid reasoning. It studies general forms that arguments take, which are valid and which are fallacies. Many people are surprised to learn how many logical fallacies abound in our culture. A common one is the ad hominem fallacy, which is the attempt to negate a claim by attaching a negative characteristic to the person making the claim. For example, if one were to argue, 'What does Bill Clinton know about strong families? He cheated on his wife', then this argument would be committing a logical fallacy, an ad hominem attack. Whatever Clinton's ideas are about strong families, they should be analyzed based on the strength of the ideas themselves. His personal life is irrelevant. Conversely, to argue that a scientist must be right because they are a scientist is to also commit the ad hominem fallacy, but in the other direction. Being who they are doesn't make their ideas any more right than anyone else's. Despite that it's reasonable to place more trust in experts, it is the expert's ideas themselves that must ultimately stand the test of truth. History has shown us that dumb people can be right and smart people can be wrong; unpopular ideas can be right and popular ideas can be wrong; laypeople can be right and authorities can be wrong. It's the idea that should ultimately be evaluated, not the person conveying it.

Logic emphasizes that conclusions hinge on the strength of their premises, facts, and interpretations. Since conclusions require foundational knowledge, reasonable arguments can be made according to the intersectional knowledge. For example, a logical framework that applies human evolution to nutrition goes like this:

Our ancestors are organisms that evolved to particular ecological niches. They ate certain types of foods available in the wild for millions of years. Due to the pressure to survive on these foods and the significant amount of time involved, evolution teaches us that our species must be well-adapted to consume these types of foods. Conversely, we are not well-adapted to foods introduced relatively recently to the human diet that first came with the dawn of agriculture about 10,000 years ago and were popularized throughout the rise of civilization thereafter, most notably after the Industrial Revolution that began ~300 years ago.

Humans have been eating certain types of food at a scale of prodigious magnitude longer than other, newer foods that were introduced after humans invented farming, animal husbandry, and food processing methods. Over vast lengths of time, natural selection can achieve an amazing degree of subtlety, allowing even small, nuanced adaptations to make their way into the genetic material of a species if the genetic trait offers an advantage. Food is fundamental to survival in the wild, so it stands to reason that the types of foods available in the environment would be the foods that humans are well-adapted to consume. This can stem back to over 25 million years ago when hominoids forged the plant-heavy gut tract that humans inherited, and to a more significant degree includes the subsequent shift in the importance of animal foods during the rise of Homo ~2.4 million years ago, all the way to the first anatomically modern humans 200,000 years ago, up to the rise of civilization a mere 10,000 years ago, and to today.

On the other hand, we are not well-adapted to consume foods that entered the human diet relatively recently with the rise of civilization, especially those that came about after the Industrial Revolution. These

Neolithic foods include things like processed flours, refined sugar, hydrogenated vegetable oils, refined salt, grains, legumes, synthetic trans fats, and corn derivatives. Ready for what science says about all these?

Refined carbohydrates contribute to heart disease and obesity.[19] [20] [21] Refined sugar has been identified as an addictive substance,[22] and a source of obesity,[23] diabetes,[24] hypertension,[25] tooth decay,[26] and heart disease.[27] Vegetable oils, rife with omega-6 fats, have been shown to disturb the body's natural omega 3:6 ratio, which heightens inflammation and oxidation.[28] In fact, in one study, replacing saturated fat with an omega-6 fatty acid increased death from all causes, coronary heart disease, and cardiovascular disease.[29]

[19] Siri-Tarino et al (2010). Saturated fat, carbohydrate, and cardiovascular disease. *American Journal of Clinical Nutrition* 91(3):502-9.

[20] Frank B (2010). Are refined carbohydrates worse than saturated fat? *American Journal of Clinical Nutrition* 91 (6): 1541-42.

[21] Jakobsen et al (2010). Intake of carbohrates compared with intake of saturated fats and myocardial infarction: importance of glycemic index. *American Journal of Clinical Nutrition* 91 (6): 1764-68.

[22] Burger and Stice (2011). Variability in reward responsivity and obesity: evidence from brain imaging studies. *Current Drug Abuse Reviews* 4(3): 182-189.

[23] Stanhope et al (2009). Consuming fructose-sweetened, not glucose-sweetened, beverages increases visceral adiposity and lipids and decreases insulin sensitivity in overweight/obese humans. *Journal of Clinical Investigation* 119(5): 1322–1334.

[24] Malik et al (2011). Sugar-sweetened beverages and risk for metabolic syndrome and type 2 diabetes. *Diabetes Care* 33 (11): 2477-2483.

[25] Chen et al (2010). Reducing consumption of sugar-sweetened beverages is associated with reduced blood pressure: a prospective study amongst United States adults. *Circulation* 121: 2398-2406.

[26] Adler et al (2013). Sequencing ancient calcified dental plaque shows changes in oral microbiota with dietary shifts of the Neolithic and Industrial revolutions. *Nature Genetics* [ePub] Retrieved from http://www.nature.com/ng/journal/vaop/ncurrent/full/ng.2536.html

[27] Lustig, Robert. (2009). "Sugar: the Bitter Truth." [Video file lecture, UCTelevision]. Retrieved from http://www.youtube.com/watch?v=dBnniua6-oM

[28] Gaubre-Eghaziber et al (2008). Nutritional intervention to reduce the n-6/n-3 fatty acid ratio increases adiponectin concentration and fatty acid oxidation in healthy subjects. *European Journal of Clinical Nutrition* 62 (11): 1287-93.

[29] Ramsden et al (2013). Use of dietary linoleic acid for secondary prevention of coronary heart disease and death: evaluation of recovered data from Sydney Diet Heart Study and updated meta-

Other human inventions like trans fat[30] and high fructose corn syrup[31] are commonly known to be harmful to the human body. Why do so many Neolithic foods appear to be detrimental to human health?

Only evolution explains this. Had any of these foods been a part of the vast timeline of human evolution, we would have evolved the ability to consume them more safely, because of the survival pressures to do so in the wild. Civilization does not afford these pressures. Neolithic foods don't have the ancient heritage of wild foods and as such were not a significant part of human evolution. Thus, evolution is the only logical explanation for understanding why industrialized foods are generally a poor choice to natural ones.

To put the question another way: why are vegetables healthy? Here is where nutritionists have done a great job. They've told us that vegetables are healthy because they are natural, full of fiber, and contain vitamins and minerals. But this only tells us *that* vegetables are good for us and fails to fully explain *why*. Only evolution tells us why.

When you think of a species that inherited a gut tract from an herbivore, suddenly vegetables make a lot of sense. Human ancestors have been eating plant foods available in the wild for millions and millions of years. It is the adaptation to this ecological environment that makes vegetables work for us today. No other explanation reaches this depth of understanding. Thus, vegetables provide a great example of how evolution serves as a logical framework within which to embed scientific (in this case, nutritional) knowledge.

After reading that long list of scientific references, some people might accuse me of cherry-picking information, only looking at the science that

---

analysis. *BMJ* 346: e8707.

[30] Food and nutrition board, institute of medicine of the national academies (2005). *Dietary Reference Intakes for Energy, Carbohydrate, Fiber, Fat, Fatty Acids, Cholesterol, Protein, and Amino Acids (Macronutrients)*. National Academies Press.

[31] Alleva and Tordoff (1990). Effect of drinking soda sweetened with aspartame or high-fructose corn syrup on food intake and body weight. *The American Journal of Clinical Nutrition*. Volume 51(6): 963-969.

supports my radical idea that evolution is relevant to health. And the truth is, they're partly right. I could have just as easily cited studies that supported the opposite of what I'm arguing about natural foods. To be sure, there are studies out there showing that milk is safe, grains are healthy, and that refined sugar can be part of a well-balanced diet. So what gives?

The difference is that those studies do not fit a logical framework; they do not fit the logic of evolution. An evolutionary paradigm provides the solid foundation for us to structure our scientific concepts, which are inherently complex and difficult to navigate, even with the support of scientific data. We can embed our science more safely and more reasonably within a logical framework than we can without one, thus fulfilling Darwin's dictum. In truth, evolution is the only valid paradigm in nutrition because it is the only idea in biology big enough to work. It is the only structure strong enough to stand. And there are no viable alternatives. Not one. So in that we have evolution, we are lucky.

Neolithic Evolution

Most people easily understand how foods introduced after the industrial revolution can be unhealthy, but what about after the agricultural revolution? Have we evolved to eat Neolithic foods over the last 10,000 years since the rise of civilization?

Yes and no. There are many examples of adaptations that arose during the last 10,000 years;[32] however, many of them are bad traits and the good ones are only partially evolved. New genetic evidence demonstrates how civilization affects the evolutionary process itself by changing the pressures of natural selection. Geneticists now understand that most of the genetic variation that exists today was introduced to the human genome mostly during the population explosion over the last 400 generations, when the rise

---

[32] Zuk, Marlene. *Paleofantasy.* WW Norton, 2013.

of civilization accelerated.[33] In one study, 86% of harmful mutations (like those contributing to disease) appear to have arisen during the Neolithic era, the last 10,000 years.[34] This means that adaptive genetic mutations (good traits) are not necessarily being selected for in the context of civilization, and maladaptive mutations (bad traits) are not necessarily being selected against, because humans no longer rely on natural environments to survive. Civilization makes it much easier to survive, so problematic genes are likely to stay in our genome, and helpful genes, like the ones that would adapt to a Neolithic lifestyle, are less likely to be selected.

Hence, the concept of natural selection, as we understand it to mean in the context of the wild, is not fully applicable to the environment of civilization. Instead, civilization sees a kind of semi-natural selection, where successful genes are not strictly chosen by the natural environment, but rather, by the pressures of the civilization itself. This leaves us with a slightly different evolutionary mechanism that fits easily with its sister concepts, artificial selection (evolution guided by the hand of humans) and natural selection (evolution guided by the hand of nature in the wild). This new concept that I call 'semi-natural selection' is taken to mean: evolution guided by the hand of civilization. It refines the idea of Neolithic evolution and helps us to understand how drastically the evolutionary pressures have changed over the last 10,000 years.

But didn't we evolve over the last 10,000 years, too? And doesn't that help tolerate a modern lifestyle? New genetic understanding weakens this argument. There is some evidence of adaptive Neolithic evolution, such as in the example of lactase persistence in milk-producing populations and skin color polymorphisms (part of what we call 'race') that are commonly believed to have arisen according to latitude and UVB sun exposure. Unfortunately,

---

[33] Keinan and Clark (2012). Recent explosive human population growth has resulted in an excess of rare genetic variants. *Science* 336 (6082): 740-743.

[34] Fu et al (2012). Analysis of 6,515 exomes reveals the origin of most human protein-coding variants. *Nature* [ePub ahead of print] Retrieved from http://www.nature.com/nature/journal/vaop/ncurrent/full/nature11690.html

milk-drinking populations still get milk-related diseases, like cancer,[35] [36] suggesting that lactase persistence, as a partial adaptation, does not protect against such incidences. And changes in skin color occurred rather recently according to genetic evidence.[37] [38] [39] It probably changed thanks to a poor diet via agriculture, which increased the importance of sunlight once vitamin D-rich animal foods in the diet declined.[40] Hence, most of the strongest examples of Neolithic evolution are not fully formed adaptations, and they tend to be isolated to small populations; therefore, they are not generally applicable to all people. Additionally, most traits that are cited were pre-existing before civilization and then mutated after civilization (e.g. extended timeline for milk tolerance). This is wholly different than an altogether new trait appearing. Even if natural selection were a fully applied process in the context of civilization as it was in the wild (which it isn't), 10,000 years is still just a short chapter in the long story of human evolution.

There's also the obvious: society's problems. If we were evolved to tolerate a Neolithic lifestyle, then why is our society rife with degenerative disease, mental health issues, and nearly ubiquitous personal anguish — all things that do not exist for the many hunter-gatherers alive today nor our Paleolithic ancestors of the past, despite the challenging conditions in which they live and lived. The takeaway here is that the human genome is ancient. It formed over millions of years according to life in the wild. This is the truth worth leveraging to our advantage.

---

[35] Ursin et al (1990). Milk consumption and cancer incidence: a Norwegian prospective study. *British Journal of Cancer* 61 (3): 456-459.

[36] Qin et al (2009). Milk consumption is a risk factor for prostate cancer: Meta-analysis of case-control studies. *Nutrition and Cancer* 48 (1): 22-27.

[37] Voight et al (2006). A Map of Recent Positive Selection in the Human Genome. *PLoS Biology* 4:72.

[38] Sabeti et al (2002). Detecting Recent Positive Selection in the Human Genome from Haplotype Structure. *Nature* 419:832-7.

[39] Gibbons, A. (2007). American Association of Physical Anthropologists Meeting. European Skin Turned Pale Only Recently, Gene Suggests. *Science* 316: 364.

[40] Lifextension. How High Latitudes and Poor Diets Turned Populations White. [Web] Retrieved from http://archaeonova.blogspot.com/2013/05/myths-of-paleo-part-two-pale-skin-in.html

Understanding Disease in Evolutionary Context

There are many diseases that exist in the wild. These diseases can be transmitted through insect bites, preparation and consumption of contaminated flesh, wounds inflicted by animals, and sharing stagnant waters with animals.[41] They tend to be viral, fungal, or bacterial in nature, and do in fact appear in the wild. After all, they are themselves evolved organisms playing the game of survival and reproduction, just like we are. However, it's vitally important to distinguish these pathogens that spur infectious disease from degenerative diseases that are not common in the wild yet are common in Western society.

The diseases of civilization, the ones that truly ravage the human population, do not significantly appear in the wild. There are traditional hunter-gatherer populations today living in harsh conditions. They die younger than modern industrialized populations because they lack access to medicine, ample food supply, sanitation, etc., but comparatively, and in spite of the apparent comforts and advancements of modern society, we civilized persons are rife with disease — including cancer, heart disease, obesity, diabetes, depression, acne, asthma, and countless other chronic, genetic, psychological, and autoimmune disorders.

These are commonly referred to as 'diseases of civilization' or 'diseases of affluence', and *they are extremely rare* in isolated hunter-gatherer populations.[42 43 44] So rare, in fact, that we should take heed. The almost complete lack of disease in hunter-gatherers is often attributed to lifestyle factors, including a diet of natural foods, balanced exercise, adequate sleep,

---

[41] Guegan et al. "Global spatial patterns of infectious diseases and human evolution." In [Stearns and Koella, Eds.] *Evolution in Health and Medicine.* New York: Oxford University Press, 2008.

[42] Price, Weston A. *Nutrition and Physical Degeneration.* Paul B. Hoeber, 1939.

[43] Cordain et al (2002). Acne vulgaris: a disease of Western civilization. *Archives of Dermatology* 138 (12): 1584-90

[44] Milton, K (2000). Hunter-gatherer diets: a different perspective. *American Journal of Clinical Nutrition* 71 (3): 665-667.

social connection, etc. But why they lack western diseases only makes sense in the light of evolution. These populations are living by the laws of nature. They highlight that it is the discordance between our evolved traits and contemporary lifestyles that leads to the general deterioration of well-being.[45]

[46] [47] [48] This is the *discord hypothesis* (or *mismatch hypothesis*) that has become so important to understanding modern disease and human well-being.

The wild has interesting clues as to the baseline potential for human health. For instance, cancer is rare in the wild (the parts untouched by human industry). On the other hand, domesticated and captive animals, including pets at home and animals in the zoo, commonly develop diseases of civilization — often the same ones as humans![49] After all, in scientific terms, humans are a self-domesticated species. (Humans are not the only ones. The well-studied example of the bonobo highlights how others species in the wild are taking strides toward self-domestication as well.)[50] The link between disease and domestication is strong, and inevitably begs the question as to why. Why are domesticated animals (including humans) more prone to disease than wild ones? Evolution answers this question and more like it: Do giraffes have neck pain? Are bald eagles scared of heights? Are night owls sleep deprived?

Stanford University neurobiologist and primatologist Robert Sapolsky touts a parallel idea in his popular science book, *Why Zebras Don't Get Ulcers*. In this work, Sapolsky covers the biology behind stress and how it causes mental

[45] Konner and Eaton (2010). Paleolithic Nutrition: 25 Years Later. *Nutrition in Clinical Practice* 25 (6): 594-602.

[46] Grinde, B (2009). Can the concept of discords help us find the causes of mental disease? *Medical Hypotheses* 73: 106-109.

[47] Booth, Chakravarthy, and Spangenburg (2004). Exercise and gene expression: physiological regulation of the human genome through physical activity. *Physiology* 543 (2): 399-411.

[48] Chakravarthy and Booth (2004). Eating, exercise, and "thrifty" genotypes: connecting the dots toward an evolutionary understanding of modern chronic disease. *Applied Physiology* 96 (1): 3-10.

[49] Natterson-Horowitz and Bowers. *Zoobiquity: What Animals Can Teach Us About Health and the Science of Healing.* Knopf, 2012.

[50] Hare, Wobber, and Wrangham (2012). The self-domestication hypothesis: evolution of bonobo psychology is due to selection against aggression. *Animal Behaviour* 83 (3): 573-585.

and physical damage to the human body through hormonal dysregulation. Many of the stressors he discusses that lead to disease are modern and out of line with the stresses in the ancestral environment. They include work stress and the demands of balancing life responsibilities. He concludes that the quality and quantity of modern stresses for the average person today is *chronically elevated* — compared to the environment of our ancestors — due to the demands of modern society. From an evolutionary perspective, humans are overly stressed in modern life because our ancient biological stress system is unable to cope in the environment of society.[51]

You see, stress is itself an evolved trait that was selected for by nature. In the wild, humans evolved stress mechanisms as a matter of survival. Stress not only induces the fight-or-flight response, but also plays a critical role in healing through inflammation. Stress is, therefore, not simply a bad thing. It is an important biological mechanism that plays multiple roles in the body. It was necessary for our ancestors in the wild in order to augment survivability and increase reproductive fitness. From an evolutionary perspective, stress is indeed a good thing. But our stress mechanisms evolved in a different environment than today, where many of the pressures of modern life do not exist. As Sapolsky point outs, the contemporary lifestyle taxes our evolved biological systems that regulate stress, ultimately leading to disease and decreased quality of life. Indeed, many diseases can be interpreted as the inevitable damage done by chronic stress.

This brings us back to the lessons of nature. Our biological systems are based on the course of millions of years of human evolution in the wild. Stress is merely one of the ways that our modern life is out of touch with human nature.[52] So what about the other ways that we are out of touch? Would eating more naturally heal the body? Would moving more naturally get better results and help to prevent injury? Would sleeping more naturally increase energy? Would achieving natural posture decrease back pain? What does

---

[51] Sapolsky, Robert. *Why Zebras Don't Get Ulcers.* Holt, 2004.

[52] Ruiz-Nunez et al (2013). Lifestyle and nutritional imbalances associated with Western diseases: causes and consequences of chronic systemic low-grade inflammation in an evolutionary context. *Journal of Nutritional Biochemistry* 24(7):1183-201.

evolution say about human nature as a collection of evolved traits? What are those traits, and how can we benefit from them? Hacking the human animal requires acknowledging these truths and building strategies around our life goals.

There is always the possibility that a new food source can be healthful. This has been observed in other species that discover new food sources and thrive. But a growing population of a particular species does not preclude that individuals of the population are optimally healthy or happy; rather, population growth highlights a species' reproductive and ecological success. Additionally, new food sources that augment human health would do so observably. There would be glaring indications of increased health in populations that adopted the food source, yet there is little evidence of Neolithic foods that do this. Most indications instead point to the detriment of human health as industrialized foods are adopted at the expense of natural foods.

The Logic of Real Food

I've been ecstatic to see real food rise to popularity over the last decade. Ideas about the importance of whole, natural foods are hugely important for everyone to hear. However, as an evolutionist, it is frustrating for me to hear the justifications for real food dance around the issue at heart; as a logician, it is dumbfounding for me to hear the arguments put forward; and as a English major, it is disheartening for me to see the phrase 'real food' lose all meaning. That's because every popular argument supporting real food is tantamount to arguing that 'real food is good for you because it is natural'.

This argument is invalid. In fact, it is a formally defined logical fallacy known as the Naturalistic Fallacy, which is to argue that something is good because it's natural, or something is bad because it is unnatural. We know that this is an invalid inference because there are natural things that are bad for you (e.g. hemlock) and unnatural things that are good for you (e.g. medicine).

Real food isn't good for you because it's *real*. Whole foods aren't good for you because they are *whole*. And natural foods aren't good for you because they are *natural*. Real whole natural foods are good for you because human beings adapted to foods available in the wild over millions of years. And guess what kinds of foods are available in the wild? This is the only valid logic for understanding why natural foods work in the human diet in the first place.

So the logical justification for real food can only be understood from an evolutionary perspective, but an evolutionary perspective also refines what we mean when we say 'real food'. Suddenly, sustainably grown wheat doesn't seem so natural, that biodynamically farmed soy doesn't seem so whole. Evolution shows us what kinds of foods human beings are adapted to and why. It seems the most important idea in biology has been missing from the logic of human diet until now.

I suspect that some health gurus know this, and I understand completely why they wouldn't emphasize evolution in their work. In America, 46% of people hold a creationist view of human origins, and only 40% of people trust in the science of evolution.[53] In order to maintain credibility and augment their influence, these professionals avoid emphasizing evolution in order to maximize their audience. Even though scientific organizations officially deny that evolution disproves God, there exists a zero-sum analysis of the debate in the minds of some believers. This zero-sum analysis is fundamentally flawed.

The Compatibility of Evolution and Creationism

Evolution does not disprove God, nor does it seek to. Evolutionary theory seeks only to prove evolution. It looks at the evidence and forms a valid framework for describing the nature of the world. As it turns out, most biological phenomena can only be understood from an evolutionary perspective. This bolsters evolutionary theory, but detracts little from theology.

---

[53] GALLUP poll results 2012. "Evolution, Creationism, and Intelligent Design." Retrieved from http://www.gallup.com/poll/21814/evolution-creationism-intelligent-design.aspx

Science and theology are two separate spheres of influence that are mostly independent of one another. The great mass of assertions in the diverse world of theology may seem to lack scientific confirmation, but this doesn't matter. The very nature of theology is unscientific, and exists outside the reach of science. In fact, there are only a handful of ways in which the two spheres clash over competing assertions.

For example, perhaps the most contentious religious assertion is the idea that Earth was created less than 10,000 years ago. While the Bible itself does not explicitly make this claim, many religious organizations endorse it. It flies in the face of the scientific consensus, which approximates the age of Earth at about 4.54 billion years, based on radiometric dating.[54] This particular example highlights how religious organizations hold on to assertions that vie with scientific truths. However, it also demonstrates that stubbornness about these issues matters little to the goals of theology. The age of the Earth does not disprove God, nor does it hinder the meaningful teachings of religious doctrine. Religious institutions risk little by revising their position. Over time these positions will likely evolve (like other old religious ideas that have fallen out of favor: the world being flat, Earth is the center of the universe, etc.). The true cost to societal progress is when religious populations denounce science for fear of it opposing their religious worldviews when the threat to the legitimacy of their religion is ultimately inconsequential.

Strategy: the Missing Element

The science of strategy is game theory, a branch of economics. It is the study of strategic decision-making, and has a place in many important fields: politics, war, business, and even personal life. No, especially personal life.

Much of the time, we are making moves in the game of life. Sometimes this can be a one-player game or a multi-player game, but in some sense we are seeking to gain an advantage of some kind or get tangible results — we

---

[54] Dalrymple, G. Brent. *The Age of the Earth.* Stanford University Press, 1991.

want to win the game.

Winning, in the general sense, can be superficial (getting rid of acne) or profound (living sustainably). But the range of human motivation is captured to some extent by our simple desire to do good for ourselves, our loved ones, our community, our species, and our planet (perhaps depending on our maturity level?). Within each arena that strategies develop, we juggle all kinds of conflicting messages and misleading information. But we have a strong tool in evolution, for it is an idea that brings clarity to many of our begging questions. It filters out bad ideas and strengthens good ones. It gives us a worldview to ask the right questions.

Strategy is a missing element to many logical inquiries. Many debates and discussions tend to ignore strategy as a subject relevant to decision-making. For instance, many of the discussions about food tend to center around what's healthy and what's not, as the popular book *Eat This, Not That* exemplifies well. A discussion of this kind can cite science in order to retain the validity of its assertions and it can stick to solid logical rationale in order to make conclusions and, yet, still, even with these things successfully executed, many individuals will not know exactly what to do about it. That's where strategy comes in.

We can't make strong decisions about anything unless we place science and reason within the context of our goals. With the example of food, an athlete will employ a different strategy than a diabetic. A vegetarian will employ a different strategy than a meat-eater. And all of these decisions are made regardless of what science or logic say about anything. If science and logic demonstrate that, say, chicken breast is good for you, then a vegetarian still won't choose it due to their strategy. An athlete may strategically choose fish over chicken breast in order to maximize athletic performance. Someone eating for the sake of enjoying their meal may prefer bacon to chicken breast, in order to optimize their enjoyment. All of these decisions are governed by the individual's strategy. Indeed, strategy plays a significant role in decision-making not only for food, but for nearly every lifestyle choice. You choose your food. You choose your workout. You choose how and when to sleep.

You choose your career. You choose the people around you. And all of these things profoundly affect the quality of your results, and therefore, the quality of your life.

I won't be using much game theory in this book, but I want to introduce it, because it's important to develop one's strategy. This will, of course, be based on goals, which are in turn based on values, perspectives, ideals, and attributes of the individual. This is something that forms out of self-knowledge. It can be as simple as thinking about what's important to you, or as broad as thinking about what's important to the world. Ultimately, these are bound to be positive, and to add tangibly to one's life.

There are all kinds of things that people want to win. In fact, people before me have written books about probably all of those things. So when I sat down and chose the topics worth exploring through the lens of evolution, I chose to look at what's worth exploring in general — things like vitality, fitness, romance, connection to others and to nature, life satisfaction and well-being, sustainability, and morality. These are some of the most important topics that can be seen more clearly in the light of evolution. They are an essential part of my personal values and, I hope, the values of my society. I believe that clearing up these complex issues will leave us with stronger communities, happier and healthier people, and a culture that honors the truth of human nature.

"Human beings are animals. We are sometimes monsters, sometimes magnificent, but always animals. We may prefer to think of ourselves as fallen angels, but in reality we are risen apes."

Desmond Morris

the human zoologist

CHAPTER 2

REVISITING HUMAN EVOLUTION, THE MOST IMPORTANT IDEA

Many don't fully understand just how lucky we are to be alive. I mean, think about it. Billions of years ago, there just happened to be a planet with enough water that ended up orbiting within the habitable zone of a sun stable enough to support life. Out of that planet's Hadean environment, the first ingredients of life were forged, and from the first organism sprouted the fingers of biodiversity, exploding into layers of biological complexity. Over eons of time these species waxed and waned, ebbed and flowed, undergoing mass extinctions and reviving into vast ecosystems that scattered the earth in stratified circles of ecology, forever interlinked and interdependent. Eventually, there came brains and with them consciousness. And then emotion. And then, finally, true intelligence, a trait that only our species owns.

Life on Earth likely began 3.7 billion years ago when a self-replicating molecule led to the Universal Common Ancestor of all life today.[55] Mystery shrouds the exact process under which this occurred, but it is believed that

---

[55] Doolittle, W. Ford (2000). Uprooting the tree of life. *Scientific American* 282 (6): 90–95.

this ancestor arose from simple chemical reactions that relied on the Hadean environment of the time.[56] Scientists have created amino acids, the 'building blocks of life,' under the hypothetical environments of early Earth, but many of the stages of origin theory remain an open question. One day, scientists may very well confirm origin theory in the lab by recreating its processes. Regardless, the tree of life starts here, and branches off over time through speciation (the branching off of new species) to achieve the biodiversity that is seen all over the world today.

Human beings are *homo sapiens sapiens*, and we've been around longer than you might think. That is to say, anatomically modern humans arose out of East Africa about 200,000 years ago.[57] Humans back then were nearly identical in mind and body as humans today. It will be important to recognize this as we explore ways that human lifestyles changed upon the arrival of civilization and society. As medical anthropologist S. Boyd Eaton declared, "99.99% of our genes were formed before the dawn of agriculture." Our genetic heritage is essentially the same as the hunter-gatherers of the world before the rise of civilization. Because our minds and bodies today were largely shaped in the wild before the rise of civilization, then exploring and interpreting our evolved traits, no matter the topic, will lead us to uncover truths about human nature and to reveal strategies for modern living that are rooted in the power and potential of human evolution.

Evolution is not exactly progress. The idea that our species improves over time is obsolete.[58] While evolution is often portrayed as a story of a simple cell transforming over eons into an intelligent being, the truth is that our species does not 'improve' out of its own volition. Rather, the lesson of evolution teaches the chaos of nature, defined by the environment and the dictates of survival and reproduction — and not all of these factors rely on intelligence or

---

[56] Peretó, J. (2005). Controversies on the origin of life. *Internal Microbiology* 8 (1): 23–31.

[57] Mcdougall, Brown, and Fleagle (2005). "Stratigraphic placement and age of modern humans from Kibish, Ethiopia". *Nature* 433 (7027): 733–736.

[58] Provine, W. B. "Progress in evolution and meaning in life". *Evolutionary Progress*. University of Chicago Press, 1988. pp. 49–79.

progress, per se. As we will see, civilization and society drastically changed the evolutionary environment, which changed the directions of human evolution.

So, What is Evolution?

Evolution is the process by which a species changes over time.[59] It is based on the idea that traits are passed down from one generation to another in the form of genes, which code for traits. For instance, consider how sons and daughters tend to look like one or both of their parents. This is the passing down of heritable traits, which extends well beyond the physical. Genes affect the development of the mind and body, so physical and mental traits are passed down — from bone structure and skin color to friendliness and intelligence.

However, the genes of offspring will vary slightly from their parents. This is due either to the introduction of new genes via random changes (replication errors in DNA) or the mix of genes from both parents as a result of reproduction.[60] Consider how brothers and sisters vary from one another and from their parents. The balance between the transmission of genetic material via offspring and the variation of that genetic material is at the heart of how a species evolves over vast lengths of time according to the pressures of the natural environment.

This is one mechanism of evolution known as 'natural selection', a term coined by Charles Darwin. It describes how certain heritable traits in a species will increase its odds of survival, in turn allowing it to reproduce more successfully, passing these heritable characteristics down to the next generation.[61] In this way, nature is 'selecting' certain traits to be passed down, based on the dictates of the environment and the concomitant pressures to

---

[59] Gould, Stephen Jay (2002). *The Structure of Evolutionary Theory.* Harvard University Press. pp. 1433

[60] Gregory, T. R. (2009). "Understanding Natural Selection: Essential Concepts and Common Misconceptions". *Evolution: Education and Outreach* 2 (2): 156–175.

[61] Darwin, Charles. *On the Origin of Species.* Gramercy, 1995.

survive.

Another mechanism of evolution by natural selection is 'sexual selection', another term coined by Charles Darwin. Sexual selection describes how the factors affecting one's reproductive success are likely to be carried on in a population. For instance, the ornate feathers of the peacock, which are used to attract mates, become important only for this purpose, rather than for the purposes of survival. Those peacocks with the best feathers are selected for by their mates, thus ensuring that their genes for ornate feathers are passed along. Over time, the feathers have evolved into beautiful displays of fertility despite the obvious detriment to the bird's anatomical functionality.

The Evidence for Evolution

Much of evolutionary theory is misunderstood or intentionally misconstrued. Many of its criticisms are unfounded, driven by propaganda rather than science. While there is a lot that we don't yet know about the evolution of life on Earth, you may be surprised at how much we do know. Let's quickly review, then, the solid evidence upon which this revolutionary idea is built. The following is taken from a presentation by Duke University geneticist, Mohamed Noor,[62] and is based on Jerry Coyne's seminal book, *Why Evolution is True*.

- **Transitional forms in the fossil record.** Evolutionary theory predicts that the first forms of life would be simple and subsequent forms would develop biological complexity. Of course, this is now confirmed by the fossil record. Also, the fossil record shows the transitional stages within and among species. For example, we have unearthed a feathered dinosaur, *Sinornithosaurus millenni*, that is believed to mark the split between birds and reptiles. Some lineages

---

[62] Noor, Mohammed. "Basic Principles and Evidence for Evolution". [Video file] Retrieved from Coursera at http://class.coursera.org/geneticsevolution-2012-001/lecture/8.

are also particularly detailed, such as that of the great whales. We have discovered ample fossil evidence illustrating the transition through time of these large aquatic mammals from their land-dwelling descendants over about 50-60 million years. (Ever wonder why whales spend all their time underwater yet breathe air? Evolution answers this riddle.)

- **Biogeography.** Isolated oceanic islands have insects, saltwater fish, and birds native to the nearby mainland. However, mammals, amphibians, and freshwater fish are starkly dissimilar to animals on the mainland. Since life forms naturally spread across the world, only the animals that can fly or swim to these islands are found both on the island and the mainland. The unique biodiversity of isolated island creatures supports the idea that they evolved there separately from the mainland, confined by the sea. Galapagos Island would be the most famous example, but there are many others.

- **Vestigial organs.** In one example, whales have vestigial hind limb bones that are useless for the whale, but are a genetic echo of its four-legged land-dwelling ancestors. Wisdom teeth often come with complications due to the changing structure of the human jaw as we slowly evolve to society's new diet (today's foraging societies do not have this problem).

- **Vestigial genes.** Geneticists have decoded genes in humans that do not materialize because the code is broken. Discovered genetic codes include the gene for making Vitamin C and the genes that would expand our olfactory receptors (sense of smell). Evolution teaches us that humans have lost these genes because of their decreasing importance in the ancestral environment. As our brains grew, the evolutionary pressures changed and we no longer needed these genes to survive.

- **Inefficient design.** Although there are beautifully mesmerizing examples of complex biological design in plants and animals, there are many examples of bad design. For instance, the laryngeal nerve in humans starts in our neck, flows down to our chest underneath the aorta, then back up to our larynx in our throats. It also does so in giraffes (since we share a common ancestor), despite the glaring inefficiency of this route. Bad design makes sense only in light of evolution. Bad design is understandable because of the tiny increments of change over each generation that build on the changes before them. Evolution cannot 'start over' but must work with what it has. Perhaps Neil DeGrasse Tyson said it best in a presentation on Stupid Design: "What's going on between our legs? An entertainment complex in the middle of a sewage system — no engineer would design that!"[63]

A Natural History of Mankind

The human timeline is always changing due to the nature of historical science, which differs necessarily in form from experimental science. Since experimentation is not possible in the historical context, the science of history is limited to finding ancient artifacts and deducing their place in history. The methods of historical science are thorough, rigorous, and based in academic discourse and dating technologies. As such, the facts and theories that are accepted by the consensus of historical experts are indeed the best we have in interpreting human history. Also, since claims can only be made according to evidence, then most of the timeline gets pushed back further and further as new evidence is discovered.

Let's tackle human evolution strategically by zooming in on the most important segment of time during human evolution and then zooming out to see why the peripheral timelines matter as well. This is from anthropologist Geoff Bond:

---

[63] Tyson, Neil DeGrasse. "Neil DeGrasse Tyson - Bad Design". [Video file] Retreived from http://www.youtube.com/watch?v=YCnGf37iiKU.

> We have our humanlike beginnings with East African Homo
> erectus over 1,000,000 years ago. Out of that population, Homo
> sapiens arose and existed for 190,000 years before leaving Africa
> about 60,000 years ago. This period, from over 1,000,000 years
> ago to 60,000 years ago is critical—it is our formative era. It is
> the time when the African environment forged the bodies that
> we possess today...[64]

Among timelines presented by experts, the quote above represents the
smallest period of time that demonstrates the importance of evolution to our
bodies and minds today. It is zooming in on a very specific million-year period
where humans evolved in a relatively small corner of the world. It highlights
the time from when 'genetically modern humans' arose up until our ancestors
left Africa. It also underscores the fact that our ancestors spent a significant
amount of time evolving in a particular environment, and therefore evolved
in a particular way. This narrow timeline represents the most important
period for the formation of minds and bodies. Now let's zoom out a little.

Humans are dated according to the genus (category) Homo, starting with
Homo habilis ~2.4 million years ago.[65] Homo habilis used stone tools, foraged
plants, and scavenged animal foods. Many of the elements of living in the wild
were the same for these humans as the ones in Bond's "formative era". Food
categories in the human diet were unchanged. They were still eating plants
and animals available in the wild, and were therefore adapted to those foods
that played a role in our ancestor's evolution. In fact, many characteristics
were the same. They survived in the wild, lived in social groups, were subject
to many of the same physical demands of nature, etc. This expands the early
human timeline, keeping it relevant to ancestral logic as it applies to the minds

---

[64] Bond, Geoff. *Deadly Harvest.* Square One, 2007.

[65] Stringer, C.B. (1994). "Evolution of Early Humans". In Steve Jones, Robert Martin & David
Pilbeam. *The Cambridge Encyclopedia of Human Evolution.* Cambridge: Cambridge University Press.
p. 242.

and bodies of humans today.

The idea of a formative era is crucial to understanding the discordance hypothesis, because it is the environment of this particular era that forged the "latest draft of our genome," as Melvin Konner, an early figure in evolutionary medicine, describes. Our genes, in some but not all ways, are in discord with the environment of civilization.[66] Exploring ways in which this works is the inevitable destination of the discordance hypothesis. It's important, then, that the "formative era" premise retains scientific validity.

It does so in two ways. First, the principle of a formative era is supported by anthropological evidence. Second, the Neolithic was not enough time or pressure to fully realize genetic adaptations. Health writer Paul Jaminet states,

>...the ancestral diet was probably similar in general outline for at least 2 million years: it consisted largely of meat, marrow, and plant foods collected from open woodlands and tree-spotted grasslands. There was sufficient time for new mutations to appear and rise to fixation, and then new mutations to appear and reach fixation against this new genetic background, and so on for many cycles. It is certainly possible that humanity became adapted to this (slowly changing) Paleolithic diet, and that the genetic variety introduced in the Holocene has been insufficient to destroy our fitness for a diet like that of the Paleolithic, and insufficient to make us well adapted to new Neolithic diets.[67]

The evidence and logic of human evolution illuminates how the human body, originally designed for life in the wild, has been thrown, for better or worse, into the environment of civilization. Therefore, seeking to resolve the discord is a worthy pursuit.

---

[66] Konner, M (2001). Evolution and the environment: will we adapt? *Western Journal of Medicine* 174(5): 360–361.

[67] Jaminet, P (2013). Paleofantasy and the state of ancestral science. [Web file] Retrieved from perfecthealthdiet.com/2013/03/paleofantasy-and-the-state-of-ancestral-science/

Anatomically modern humans emerged from East Africa around 200,000 years ago. However, we can refine this idea by exploring the emergence of *behaviorally* modern humans, about 40,000-80,000 years ago. We don't yet know why this era in particular was so special. Many theories abound, including sudden genetic mutations and volcanic winters, but it is generally agreed upon that it was during the time just before the human population expanded within and outside of Africa. During this time period, humans probably developed new cultural innovations based on new evolutionary achievements in brain, likely language, capabilities.[68] Now let's zoom out again.

In 2010, the journal Nature published a study by archaeologist Shannon McPhernon, who discovered the remains of a butchered animal dating back 3.4 million years, pre-dating humans but coinciding with the human ancestor Australopithecus afarensis.[69] This surprising new evidence pushes back the ancestral timeline for animal consumption and tool use by almost a million years, implicating that the trend for scavenging existed earlier than previously believed. Although this evidence is too new and divergent in order to reach a scientific conclusion, it is strong enough to reasonably expand the timeline of a fundamental ancestral diet back to 3.4 million years of plant and animal consumption, forging an even stronger interpretation of the importance of evolution to the formation of our bodies today.

Before the first humans, there were hominids going back over 25 million years. These were tree-dwelling primates in the forest regions of Africa. They ate heavily plant-based diets, forging the gut tract that the Homo lineage ultimately inherited — one that eventually evolved for meat-eating.[70] They reigned during the Miocene period, before the forests receded to make way for grassland savannah. It was from these hominids that we inherited bodies

---

[68] Atkinson et al (2009). Bayesian coalescent inference of major human mitochondrial DNA haplotype expansions in Africa. *Proceedings of the Royal Society* B 276: 367-73.

[69] McPherron et al (2010). Evidence for stone-tool-assisted consumption of animal tissues before 3.39 million years ago at Dikika, Ethiopia. *Nature* 466: 857–860.

[70] Milton, K (1999). A hypothesis to explain the role of meat-eating in human evolution. *Evolutionary Anthropology* 8:11–21.

and minds ready for the next stage of evolution: tool use, language, and intelligence. In fact, we are still strikingly similar to our primate cousins today.[71] This ancient history of our pre-human ancestors is relevant because it highlights many human traits that are simply echoes of our past. (We will cover many of these important features in the following chapters of the book.)

Now let's fast forward to 60,000 years ago when humans first left Africa and began to slowly populate every region of the world.[72] This was the time during when our species entered new geographies and climates, and saw some degree of differentiation, what biologists call 'polymorphism', and is part of what we refer to as 'race'.[73] While there was a great deal of differentiation in terms of adaptation to climate/environment, many important things stayed the same. Our hunter-gatherer diets, physical movements, and the dependence on social groups all still mattered for survival. Thus, throughout the timelines discussed, the wild defined the aspects of our survival, and it was this very nature to which our species evolved — all the way up to the rise of civilization.

The turn of the Neolithic and the rise of civilization are marked by the transition to farming culture, roughly estimated as having occurred 10,000 years ago.[74] However, the advent of cultivation started a slow process of transition beginning 12,000 years ago[75] (first evidence of human farming) and did not end until reaching nearly all regions of the world 5,000 years ago.[76] Indeed, there are still some remote hunter-gatherer populations in the world

---

[71] Milton and Demment (1998). Digestive and passage kinetics of chimpanzees fed high and low fiber diets and comparison with human data. *Journal of Nutrition* 118:1.

[72] Martin, Meredith (2011). *Born in Africa: The Quest for the Origins of Human Life*. PublicAffairs. p. 148.

[73] Jablonski, Nina (2004). The Evolution of Human Skin and Skin Color. *Annual Review of Anthropology* 33: 585-623.

[74] Rindos, David (December 1987). *The Origins of Agriculture: An Evolutionary Perspective*. Academic Press.

[75] Kislev et al (2006). Early domesticated fig in Jordan valley. *Science* Vol. 312 No. 5778: 1372-1374.

[76] Ammerman, A. J. & Cavalli-Sforza, L. L. *The Neolithic Transition and the Genetics of Populations in Europe* (Princeton University Press, Princeton, New Jersey, 1984).

today that contribute to our understanding of ancient human behavior before the rise of civilization, though these populations, too, have been evolving.[77] Interestingly, the idea that hunter-gatherers simply gave up their lifestyle to begin farming has been debunked. In fact, it was the population growth of farming tribes that pushed them into new territories, displacing or meshing with other hunter-gatherers.[78] The spread of farming populations, perhaps based on their success, was the catalyst for the spread of the agrarian lifestyle.

By 4,000 years ago, a sedentary agriculture-based lifestyle had become the mainstay of the human population, yet the ample food supply paradoxically decreased human nutrition. This is supported by evidence that nutritional standards of Neolithic populations were generally poor compared to that of hunter-gatherers, and life expectancy may have in fact been shorter, in part due to diseases that were exacerbated by increased crowding. Average height, for instance, decreased from 5' 10" (178 cm) for men and 5' 6" (168 cm) for women to 5' 3" (165 cm) and 5' 1" (155 cm), respectively. It took all the way until the twentieth century for average human height to return to pre-Neolithic levels.[79] Of the newly cultivated and domesticated foods during the Neolithic transition (oats, barley, wheat, etc.) most are far less nutrient-dense compared to foods available in the wild to which our species evolved, as well as to their modern alternatives (kale, spinach, papaya, etc.). The new survival pressure to survive on Neolithic foods in an environment of civilization transformed human evolution for the next 10,000 years, all the way up to today, increasing the rate of evolution at a scale of magnitude due to the sea change in evolutionary pressure.[80] The vast change in environment, spreading human genes, and selection pressure led to the morphology of certain populations over the world and to fundamental changes in heritable characteristics.

---

[77] Cordain et al (2000). Plant-animal subsistence ratios and macronutrient energy estimations in worldwide hunter-gatherer diets. *American Journal of Clinical Nutrition* 71 (3): 682-692.

[78] Sokal et al (1991). Genetic evidence for the spread of agriculture in Europe by demic diffusion. *Nature* 351: 143-145.

[79] Shermer, Michael (2001). *The Borderlands of Science*. Oxford University Press, 2001: p. 250.

[80] Cochran and Harpending. *The 10,000 Year Explosion*. Basic Books, 2009.

And then came the most potent historical event that affects our lives today. It was itself the product of evolved intelligence and the shifting dynamics of civilization, a sign of human ingenuity and progress: the Industrial Revolution. With it came the mechanization of labor that enabled economies of scale at magnitudes before unseen. Pioneers of industry were able to efficiently produce and alter goods for the marketplace, which in turn lowered cost for consumers. Western culture changed in almost every way imaginable. Economic prosperity led to further development of the modes of production and, suddenly, the modern lifestyle was born. With it came the fueling of dense city centers, the birth of the nuclear family, and shifting cultural ideals. Importantly, out of this environment came new ways to process grains, refine sugar and salt, and store foods through canning, bottling, packaging, etc. Many of the technological advances in food processing during this era were detrimental to the human diet and to public health — physically, psychologically, and spiritually.

Human evolution tells a story of change and triumph, of turbulence and chaos. We see a species that lived a rugged yet balanced life in the wild for millions of years. Then, suddenly, that species became subject to its own evolutionary potential, developing intelligence enough to spur invention, leading to tools and practices that sparked the explosion of civilization, evolving and devolving in more ways than we know. Perhaps it is tempting to look back on the human animal in the wild before the rise of civilization and see an inferior or superior species, but the truth is that the animal of our past is more like us than we care to admit. That animal is the ghost in our genetic material, echoing in our hearts, bodies, and minds.

Genetics and Environment

For every lifeform on earth, the genotype determines the potential for each evolutionary trait. How tall, fast, smart, or social an organism will be depends on the degree to which the genotype allows those traits to foster. As E.O Wilson once said, "Genes keep culture on a leash." However, it is ultimately the environment that determines how genes manifest in reality. Scientists refer to the phenotype (genetic expressions), environment, and ontogeny (programmed development). Working together, nature and nurture are hugely influential to guiding the development of an organism.

In an open field, plants that get plenty of sunlight grow tall. If the sunlight is diminished, those same plants would not grow as tall. Just like these plants, our growth in every way depends on environmental factors. We can't do much to change our genetics, but we can control our environment, the factors and inputs that ultimately affect our genetic expression. This is what makes the environment and our culture so crucial to human well-being.

Tapping Human Potential

During the Olympic games, I can't help but rejoice in the spectacle of athletic achievement. Olympians pursue goals with such talent, devotion, and work ethic that to observe them in action is spellbinding. They often surpass expectations with new world records that push the boundaries of human potential. While most of us do not seek Olympic glory in our day-to-day lives, we do seek other important goals. In life, we seek the acceptance of others, physical intimacy with loved ones, vibrant energy and mental focus, some level of physical fitness, and robust immune function. We seek fun and meaning and satisfaction. All of us seek love, health, and happiness.

Living our lives, we must decide for ourselves what these things mean and what goals they ultimately become. But to reach the heart of those decisions, we must know and understand our minds and bodies. And these are best understood in the context of human evolution, using this understanding to help ourselves. As the philosopher Alain de Botton recently declared, "A culture which gives a role to guidance and the self-help book stands a chance of making at least one or two fewer mistakes than the previous generation in the time that remains."

It just means becoming better. For some, this may mean improving upon things already accepted as normal, like acne or asthma. For others, this may mean discovering new levels of happiness or the heights of love. People have chased these things before, but they have done so without a paradigm, without a unifying idea. Evolution is that powerful idea that unites the scientific disciplines, that sheds light on where we come from and who we are. It is the ultimate framework within which to build hypotheses or frame questions.

An average, normal person may say that they are "healthy," but really all they mean is that they are disease-free or comparatively able-bodied relative to their peers. Yet it is also likely that their teeth came in crooked, they have had acne for years, they have poor posture, bad eyesight, trouble sleeping, stomach aches, and overactive allergies — yet they are "healthy"! This fallacy pervades our culture, that something is 'normal, therefore good'. It is a notion that hinders human progress and limits our understanding of human nature.

An evolutionary perspective on health inevitably begs the question of optimization. If there are a set of evolved traits that all humans have inherited as a species, then given what we know about evolution, these traits must be predictable, identifiable, and optimizable. Like any system, these traits rely on certain factors. In light of evolutionary theory, we should be able to tap the potential of these systems. This is how we game the system. This is how we hack the human animal.

Reaching our potential is the ultimate goal of applying evolutionary theory strategically. It means creating a better world for ourselves and others, not only by knowing ourselves, but by knowing our species and knowing our place in the world from a big picture perspective. To understand evolution is to understand our lives, and only through understanding can we improve.

Is Our Species Getting Dumber?

It's a common tongue-in-cheek idea that civilization is causing our species to lose its average intelligence. This is based on the fossil record, which says human brain size peaked about 20,000 years ago, and the presumption that "clever people—who on average have slightly bigger brains—aren't having more babies than less-clever people."[81] There may be something to this because there turns out to be a strong correlation between intelligence and not having babies. One study, published in 2010, quantified a loss of .8 IQ points per generation in the USA.[82] Another, published in 2008, predicts a loss of 1.28 IQ points by year 2050 in the world population.[83]

Stanford biochemist Gerald Crabtree covers a similar idea in the 2012 paper "Our Fragile Intellect," which proposes that human intelligence has been in steady decline since its peak 2-6,000 years ago. His hypothesis is based on the fact that intelligence exists as a matrix of genes that are fragile to bad mutations. Since civilization creates an environment where these bad mutations are not selected against, it may be predictable that human intelligence is fading at the rate that these mutations spread throughout the population.[84] Since brain size is a heritable characteristic[85] (as well as environmental), then the average brain size *for the human population* must be getting smaller over time. To some extent, this may indicate a dumbing down of the human mind. But don't let this news alarm you, because the nature of human intelligence has changed dramatically since the days before civilization, and the future of intelligence is only promising.

Today, human knowledge is cumulative over time, due to the human institutions of writing, education, media, technology, etc. Information, wisdom, and knowledge is passed down and built upon by subsequent generations more efficiently than ever, and increasingly

---

[81] Neal, Chris Silas (May 24, 2012). "Human Evolution Isn't What it Used to Be." *Wall Street Journal*. Retrieved from http://online.wsj.com/article/SB10001424052702303610504577418511907146478.html.

[82] Meisenberg (2010). The reproduction of intelligence. *Intelligence* 38 (2): 220-230.

[83] Lynn and Harvey (2008). The decline of the world's IQ. *Intelligence* 36 (2): 112-120.

[84] Crabtree, Gerald (2012). Our fragile intellect. *Trends in Genetics* 29 (1): 1-3.

[85] Bartley, A., Jones, D., and Weinberger, D. (1997). Genetic variability of human brain size and cortical gyral patterns. *Brain* 120 (2): 257-269.

so, thanks to technology. That also means that human intelligence today is more collective. It is often working together, rather than one's individual pursuits, that leads to intellectual progress. Additionally, the structure of society yields ever-increasing efficacy in developing most (but not all) forms of intelligence. Environment counts because it changes the expression of genetic traits; for instance, doing math makes the brain better at doing math. Our math programs our clearly more challenging than math in nature, and they only continue to improve. And lastly, we have achieved strength in numbers. There are 7 billion people on Earth and counting. Compare that to less than a million people pre-civilization. The population matters because genetic diversity is more common than many realize.[86] Every person is going to be different, and some are going to be outliers on either end of the intelligence spectrum (and also in the spectrum of each form of intelligence: social, logical, kinesthetic, linguistic, etc.). That means that a larger population will have more outliers, for better or worse. In turn, these really smart people are likely to make lasting contributions to society that will live on.

But the real promise for the future of human intelligence lies in a place that many people don't like to talk about. The paper cited above, "The Decline of the World's IQ," ends its abstract with a technological hint of hope: "It is possible that the 'new eugenics' of biotechnology may evolve to counteract dysgenic fertility."

Measuring intelligence is a slippery slope. Only about half of intelligence is heritable. Even quantifying general intelligence, as psychologists do with the variable g, is a contentious topic. Despite the controversy, there is no evidence that people are getting dumber. In fact, it is widely accepted that people are getting smarter at about 3 IQ

---

[86] Novembre et al. An abundance of rare functional variants in 202 drug target genes sequenced in 14,002 people. *Science.* [Web file] Retrieved from http://www.sciencemag.org/content/early/2012/05/16/science.1217876.short

points per decade, which is referred to as the Flynn effect. Although this may appear to shown human progress, measuring these things may be slightly too difficult. As Matt Ridley points out, "The heritability of intelligence may therefore be about the genetics of nurture, just as much as the genetics of nature."[87]

The future holds almost unbelievable promise. There are already brain implants that read radio waves and translate them into action robotically. Stephen Hawking writes emails using only his mind. Michio Kaku is a theoretical physicist who predicts that memory and learning will be uploaded, much like a computer. His book, *The Future of the Mind*, deciphers the thinking brain and how it will one day run in concert with the mechanics of the future. We don't know what dreams will come, but it is conceivable that we will one day hijack the evolutionary process. His most fascinating prediction: that consciousness may one day exist outside the body, allowing humans to finally achieve immortality.

The Myth of the Caveman

Human ancestors are often believed to have lived in caves, but this is what scientists call observer bias. Many ancient artifacts are found in caves, which lead to the idea that we must have lived there. But artifacts are found in caves not because that's where humans lived. Artifacts are found in caves because caves are good environments for preserving artifacts. It should be no wonder why it's more difficult to find million-year old artifacts on coastlines or open grasslands, which are subject to the harsh elements of nature. In fact, human ancestors preferred life on the savanna or the coast. Eventually, though, they spread to nearly all areas of Earth, inhabiting even its deserts and mountains.

---

[87] Ridley, Matt. "Intelligence." *Genome*. HarperCollins, 2000. pp. 89-90.

"Technology's double punishment is to both make us age prematurely and live longer."

Nassim Taleb

economist

CHAPTER 3

A DISEASE-PROOF DIET
DEFINED BY THE WILD

Evolution helps us to understand nutrition at its most basic level: life's need to procure elements, the simple dead molecules swimming in the great mass of Earth. By necessity, organisms must procure or generate certain elementary ingredients in the recipe of life. Humans and all other life forms have evolved organ systems to do just that. We have lungs that get oxygen to our blood, a heart that circulates the nutrients in our blood throughout the body, skin that harvests vitamin D from sunlight, and a digestive system that plays a central role in getting most of what we need from food by breaking it down and absorbing it. So eating a banana for potassium, for example, is serving the same purpose as taking a breath of fresh air for oxygen. Life requires these ingredients, and our organ systems have developed to acquire and manage them in the maintenance of life. This is the evolutionary legacy of food, the very reason why we even need it in the first place.

The next crucial concept that many overlook in the diet debate is another fact of evolution: that organisms adapt to ecological niche(s) as a matter of survival. Therefore, food helps to define a species. The anteater eats ants not because it happens to like ants, but because ants represented a food source that anteaters were especially suited to exploiting. As the ancestors of the anteater exploited this food source over eons of time, their descendants became more and more specialized to this purpose until it became a defining characteristic of this particular animal.

Evolution helps us safely predict and assume certain things about ants in the anteater diet, and rodents in the snake diet, and nuts in the squirrel diet, and all of these predictions and assumptions are greatly important to understanding human nutrition. We can predict that the anteater diet provides adequate nutrition to meet the needs of the anteater. We can predict that rodents help the snake find an optimal, though compromised, point of health and well-being. And we can predict that nuts in the squirrel diet do not significantly contribute to squirrel disease. See where I'm going with this?

Using the tenets of evolution, we can predict a natural diet for *Homo sapiens*, a healthy diet for humans, simply by examining the ecological niches of human ancestors, because it is a biological certainty that the human genome is adapted, however perfectly or imperfectly, to the types of foods available in those niches. This is the profound truth about diet that can only be seen clearly in the light of evolution.

A natural history of human diet illustrates a species whose ancestors ate food available in the wild. To a significant degree, people within this time frame lived on certain types of plant and animal foods.[88] Evolution teaches us that our species must then be well-adapted to consume these types of foods, due to the survival pressure to do so and the extensive length of time involved. Of particular importance is identifying modern versions of these types of foods and developing a strategy for maximizing their potential.

Conversely, we are likely not fully adapted to consume new foods that entered the human diet relatively recently after the dawn of agriculture and especially after the Industrial Revolution.[89] The explosion of the human

---

[88] Richards, Michael P. (2002). A brief review of the archaeological evidence for Palaeolithic and Neolithic subsistence. *European Journal of Clinical Nutrition* 56 (12): 1270–78.

[89] Lindeberg et al (2003). "Biological and Clinical Potential of a Palaeolithic Diet". *Journal of Nutritional and Environmental Medicine* 13 (3): 149–60.

population after the turn of the Neolithic is due to many factors. One important aspect of the post-industrial society was increased survivability based on ample food supply. Therefore, evolution throughout the Neolithic era may have decreased the evolutionary pressure of survival based on food resources. This, in turn, would have led to insufficient pressure to alter the genotypic norms of the population in regard to modern foods, thus decreasing the extent (and even the potential) to which we are evolved to these foods.

The vast majority of our genome is evolved to a pre-agricultural lifestyle, and the introduction of new foods may spur the development of modern diseases, often called the 'diseases of civilization' or the 'diseases of affluence'.[90] A 2002 paper entitled "Evolutionary Health Promotion" presents the validity of an evolutionary paradigm to the medical establishment:

> ...shortcomings [in medicine] may reflect lack of an overall conceptual framework, a deficiency that might be corrected by adopting evolutionary premises: (1) The human genome was selected in past environments far different from those of the present. (2) Cultural evolution now proceeds too rapidly for genetic accommodation—resulting in dissociation between our genes and our lives. (3) This mismatch between biology and lifestyle fosters development of degenerative diseases.[91]

While calling for further study through the lens of evolution, these researchers point out that many of the lifestyle factors of today are out of line with the way that humans evolved. Consider the popularization of grain farming as recently as 5-10,000 years ago. Is that enough time for our species to evolve for its consumption? According to organic chemist Mathieu LaLonde, it is not:

---

[90] Cordain et al (2005). Origins and evolution of the western diet: health implications for the 21st century. *Journal of Clinical Nutrition* 81(2): 341-354.

[91] Eaton et al (2002). Evolutionary health promotion. *Preventive Medicine* 34(2): 109-118.

There's been insufficient time and insufficient evolutionary pressure for complete adaptation to seed consumption to arise in *Homo sapiens* and as a result, individuals that tolerate grains and legumes should be considered the minority, not the majority.[92]

In this argument, both the *time* of evolution is noted, as well as the *pressure* of evolution to influence the heritable characteristics of a population. During the chaotic rise of civilization over the last 10,000 years (really the last 5,000 years and especially the last 200 years), neither of these requirements were met for nature to sufficiently select for genetic traits that effectively process Neolithic foods.

This isn't to say that cultivated cereal grains are therefore maladaptive. Traditional agrarian cultures consume varying amounts of whole grains (and legumes), prepared traditionally, without suffering from many of the diseases of civilization.[93] However, dietary sensitivity to cereal grains, particularly to wheat, is hard to detect yet surprisingly common.[94][95] Wheat is increasingly implicated in a range of diseases. It's implicated in brain disorders,[96] in nearly every inflammatory skin disease,[97] in non-celiac bowel diseases,[98] and in the

---

[92] EvolutionTV. Mat LaLonde: The Science Behind the Paleolithic Diet. [Video file] Retrieved from http://www.youtube.com/watch?feature=player_embedded&v=bmL0gKEz00Q.

[93] Miller, Daphne. *The Jungle Effect: Healthiest Diets From Around the World.* William Morrow Paperbacks, 2009.

[94] Hadjivassiliou et al (2010). Gluten sensitivity: from gut to brain. *The Lancet Neurology* 9(3):318-330.

[95] Carroccio et al (2012). Non-celiac wheat sensitivity diagnosed by double-blind placebo-controlled challenge: exploring a new clinical entity. *American Journal of Gastroenterology* [ePub ahead of print] Retrieved from http://www.ncbi.nlm.nih.gov/pubmed/22825366.

[96] Volta and De Giorgio (2009). Gluten sensitivity: an emerging issue behind neurological impairment? *Lancet Neurology* 9(3): 233-235.

[97] Marzano et al (2012). Interactions between inflammation and coagulation in autoimmune and immune-mediated skin disease. *Current Vascular Pharmacology [as of yet unprinted].*

[98] Biesiekierski et al (2012). Gluten causes gastrointestinal symptoms in patients without celiac disease: a randomized double-blind controlled trial. *American Journal of Gastroenterology* 106(3): 508-14.

matrix of insulin resistance, inflammation, and body fat accumulation.[99] In fact, normal people are documented experiencing an inflammatory response to wheat, which hints at toxicity in humans.[100] And it makes perfect sense in the light of evolution. A 2012 paper states,

> Possibly the introduction of gluten-containing grains, which occurred about 10,000 years ago with the advent of agriculture, represented an evolutionary challenge that created the conditions for human diseases related to gluten exposure...[101]

And lastly, grains are nutritionally inferior to their wild alternatives (fruits, veggies, tubers),[102] which humans have been eating for millions of years — all of which contain less toxins to boot. Therefore, it is both reasonable and strategic to adopt a diet that replaces cereal grains with more nutrient-dense, toxin-free forms of carbohydrate, such as fruits, starchy vegetables, and tubers.

The Light of Evolution

The importance of an evolutionary perspective to human health has been championed by experts and academics alike. In January, 2008, evolutionary biologists Randolph Neese and Stephen Stearns from the University of Michigan and Yale University published a resonant call to the health fields in a

---

[99] Soares et al (2012). Gluten-free diet reduces adiposity, inflammation, and insulin resistance associated with the induction of PPAR-alpha and PPAR-gamma expression. *Journal of Nutritional Biochemistry* (12) 00226-4.

[100] Bernardo et al (2007). Is gliadin really safe for non-coeliac individuals? Production of interleukin 15 in biopsy culture from non-coeliac individuals challenged with gliadin peptides. *Gut* 56 (6): 889-890.

[101] Sapone et al (2012). Spectrum of gluten related disorders: consensus on new nomenclature and classification. *BMC Medicine* 10 (13).

[102] Vanderhoof, J. (1998). Immunonutrition: the role of carbohydrates. *Nutrition* 14: 595.

paper titled, "The Great Opportunity: Evolutionary Applications to Medicine and Public Health," where they state:

> The canyon between evolutionary biology and medicine is wide... Some evolutionary technologies, such as population genetics, serial transfer production of live vaccines, and phylogenetic analysis, have been widely applied. Other areas, such as infectious disease and aging research, illustrate the dramatic recent progress made possible by evolutionary insights. In still other areas, such as epidemiology, psychiatry, and understanding the regulation of bodily defenses, applying evolutionary principles remains an open opportunity. In addition to the utility of specific applications, an evolutionary perspective fundamentally challenges the prevalent but fundamentally incorrect metaphor of the body as a machine designed by an engineer. Bodies are vulnerable to disease – and remarkably resilient – precisely because they are not machines built from a plan. They are, instead, bundles of compromises shaped by natural selection in small increments to maximize reproduction, not health. Understanding the body as a product of natural selection, not design, offers new research questions and a framework for making medical education more coherent. [103]

The call for health professionals to include evolution in their understanding of human biology is a strategy that may seem obvious. However, as the authors of this study note, most medical professionals don't understand evolution in depth, and most medical schools don't have evolutionary biologists on their faculty. The authors choose interesting words to describe our "machine"-like bodies, built from "a plan" or "design," a subtle accusation that medicine is

---

[103] Nesse, R. M. and Stearns, S. C. (2008). The great opportunity: Evolutionary applications to medicine and public health. *Evolutionary Applications* 1: 28–48.

built on archaic perspectives rather than contemporary scientific ones. Evolution should be recognized for its fundamental role in biology and, by extension, medicine, an establishment highly resistant to change. We are part of an era/movement/paradigm-shift that will fill the "gap" between human nature and public health, one that has been closed to some degree over the last decade with the rise of Darwinian Medicine, Evolutionary Psychology, and Ancestral Health.

And it's about time. The idea was first introduced by — you guessed it — Charles Darwin in 1794 when he wrote *On the Origin of Species*, noting that an evolutionary perspective may help to "unravel the theory of diseases." But the first nutritional anthropology didn't take place until the early 1930s when Audrey Richards studied African tribes in Zambia.[104] Perhaps the most popular work connecting Western disease to Western lifestyle arose in 1939 when dentist-turned-anthropologist Weston A. Price published his research regarding "primitive" cultures around the world, looking to reveal the sources of their robust health.[105] Traditional cultures that Price studied ate foods close to nature. These populations were relatively disease-free and of generally superior health than westerners (taller, stronger, teeth came in straight — wisdom teeth too — and virtually no psychological disorders), implicating the western lifestyle not only in the development of physical disease but also in contributing to the detriment of overall health.

The current movement to allow evolution to inform us about food may have first been popularized by gastroenterologist Walter Voegtlin in 1975 with the publication of the book, *The Stone Age Diet*, which was based on human ecology and evolution, as well as his success healing gut-related problems for his patients with a diet inspired by the story of human evolution. Then in 1981, Hubert Trowell and Denis Burkit compiled an impressive amount of research in a book about hunter-gatherers and primitive agriculturalists around the world, noting throughout that industrialization,

---

[104] Raymond Firth (1985). "Audrey Richards 1899-1984." *Man* 20(2): 341-344.

[105] Price, Weston A. *Nutrition and Physical Degeneration*. New York, London: Paul B. Hoeber, 1939.

urbanization, and westernization commonly increased rates of the diseases of civilization.[106] In addition, a group of scientists published a paper in the New England Journal of Medicine in 1985 that states, "Natural selection has provided us with nutritional adaptability; however, human beings today are confronted with diet-related health problems."[107] Then in 1989, those same scientists, Boyd Eaton, Marjorie Shostak, and Melvin Konner, all MDs or PhDs or both, wrote a book compiling some of their research about the evolutionary implications for health, laying out guidelines for healthy living that mimicked the Paleolithic model.[108] Note that it was only once every few years that academia even explored these topics, despite their obvious relationship to public health.

This first experimental science that directly tested evolutionary eating adaptations did not occur until 1984.[109] It was a study performed by Dr. Kerin O'Dea of the University of Melbourne and published in the journal *Diabetes*. Ten middle-aged Australian aborigines, all originally born and raised in the outback, had lived their early days as hunter-gatherers, learning the skills necessary to survive, until they were ultimately forced to settle in a rural part of western Australia exposed to Western foods. Predictably, all of them developed type-2 diabetes. O'Dea asked these aborigines to return to their hunter-gatherer lifestyle for seven weeks. They agreed, travelling back to the land from which they originated. They ate kangaroos, birds, crocodiles, turtles, shell fish, yams, figs, crayfish, freshwater bream, and bush honey. At experiment's end, average weight lost was 16.5 pounds, blood cholesterol dropped 12%, and triglycerides diminished a whopping 72%. Due to the lack of control, there may have been confounding factors and unclear conclusions as to the cause of their improved health; nevertheless, the results were astonishing.

---

[106] Trowell and Burkit. *Western Diseases: Their Emergence and Prevention.* Edward Arnold, 1981.

[107] Eaton and Konner (1985). Paleolithic nutrition: a consideration of its nature and current implications. *The New England Journal of Medicine* 312 (5): 283-289.

[108] Eaton, Shostak, and Konner. *The Paleolithic Prescription.* HarperCollins, 1989.

[109] O'Dea, K. (1984). Marked improvement in carbohydrate and lipid metabolism in diabetic Australian aborigines after temporary reversion to traditional lifestyle. *Diabetes* 33(6):596-603.

There wasn't a modern experiment testing ancestral diets until 2007. In this study, 29 patients with type-2 diabetes and heart disease were placed on either a Paleolithic-style diet (veggies, fruits, meat, fish) or a Mediterranean diet (whole grains, margarine, low-fat dairy, veggies, fruits, fish, oils). After 12 weeks on either diet, blood glucose tolerance (a risk factor for heart disease) improved in both groups, but was better in the Paleolithic dieters. In the author's own words: "...avoiding Western foods is more important than counting calories, fat, carbohydrate or protein."[110]

In 2007, Dr. Osterdahl in the department of neurobiology at Sweden's Karolinska Institute conducted a study by putting 14 healthy subjects on a Paleolithic diet. After only three weeks, the subjects lost weight, reduced their waist size, and saw significant reductions in blood pressure and plasminogen activator inhibitor (a substance in blood which promotes clotting and accelerates artery clogging). No control group was used in this pilot study, so some will argue that the benefits may not necessarily be due to the diet. However, better controlled more recent experiments show similar results.

In 2009, an outstanding study by Dr. Frassetto of the University of California, San Francisco put nine inactive subjects on a Paleolithic diet for a mere 10 days. The diet was exactly matched in calories with the subjects' usual diet, eliminating the possibility of the confounding factor of calorie-cutting. Any beneficial changes in the subjects' health could not be related to reductions in calories, but rather to changes in the kinds of foods eaten. Out of the participants on the paleo diet, either eight or all nine of them saw improvements in blood pressure, arterial function, insulin, total cholesterol, LDL cholesterol, and triglycerides. This study is remarkable due to the rapid improvement in health markers for each and every patient after only ten days.[111]

A recent scientific experiment directly testing the Paleolithic diet was

---

[110] Lindeberg et al (2007). A Palaeolithic diet improves glucose tolerance more than a Mediterranean-like diet in individuals with ischaemic heart disease. *Diabetologia* 50(9):1795-1807.

[111] Frassetto et al (2009). Metabolic and physiologic improvements from consuming a Paleolithic, hunter-gatherer type diet. *European Journal of Clinical Nutrition* 63(8): 947-955.

conducted in 2009 by Dr. Jonsson and associates at Lund University, Sweden. Thirteen patients with type-2 diabetes were assigned a Paleolithic diet for 3 months, and then the same 13 patients were assigned a diabetes diet as recommended by the dietary guidelines for a second period of 3 months. The diabetes diet was intended to reduce total fat by increasing whole grain bread and cereals, low fat dairy products, fruits, and vegetables — and at the same time, restricting animal foods. Conversely, the Paleolithic diet was lower in grains, dairy, potatoes, beans, and baked foods, but higher in fruits, vegetables, meat, and eggs compared to the diabetes diet. The cross-over design was an important control for the experiment. The same 13 people doing two 3-month periods of dieting. This made the data more reliable. Compared to the diabetes diet, the paleo diet resulted in improved weight loss, waist size, blood pressure, HDL cholesterol, triglycerides, blood glucose, and hemoglobin A1c (a marker for long term blood glucose control). This experiment represents the most powerful example to date of the effectiveness of eating according to the tenets of evolution, and of the enormous potential for treating people with debilitating health problems.[112] This study was later analyzed to conclude that a Paleolithic-style diet is more satiating per calorie than even a Mediterranean diet.[113]

Evolutionary applications are overdue, and the work that has been done is barely scratching the surface of its potential. Evolution and diet are obviously related, which is something that has been thoroughly covered.[114] [115] It was a natural diet that made us human, and only evolution illuminates what that diet is. So where does that leave us? Why has it taken so long to get behind these ideas?

---

[112] Jonsson et al (2009). Beneficial effects of a Paleolithic diet on cardiovascular risk factors in type 2 diabetes: a randomized cross-over pilot study. *Cardiovascular Diabetology* 8:35.

[113] Jonsson et al (2010). A Paleolithic diet is more satiating per calorie than a mediterranean-like diet in individuals with ischemic heart disease. *Nutrition and Metabolism* 7:85.

[114] SB Eaton (1996). An evolutionary perspective enhances understanding of human nutritional requirements. *Journal of Nutrition* 126: 1732-40.

[115] Teaford and Ungar (2000). Diet and the evolution of the earliest human ancestors. *PNAS* 97: 13506-11.

Reasons abound why academia would be resistant to the interpretation of evolution in health. Evolution is an idea that has been stained by the course of history. Skeptics fear it will fuel racism, sexism, anti-theism, hierarchy, and even encroach on animal rights. The establishments that haven't yet adopted evolution as a fundamental principle of their practices — namely, medicine, public health, psychology, and nutrition — are the final frontier where the ideas of evolution will improve the worldviews, methodologies, and results of each establishment. It will lead to the exploration of more potent hypotheses. It will lead to the abandonment of flawed conventional wisdoms. Ultimately, it will drastically improve the dynamics of public health, and lead to better lives for all. This is the truth of evolution, the promise of a renewed idea.

The Ancestral Health Movement

Everyone wants their food to be 'natural' because everyone understands the power of nature. But nature can only be understood in evolutionary terms. And in the of light of evolution, even seemingly positive buzz-words like, "all-natural feedlot beef" and "organic whole wheat pasta" are not 'natural' or 'organic' to the human diet. The things that are truly natural to the human diet must fit an evolutionary perspective. Indeed, evolution sheds light on nearly every aspect of human nature. Recently, many people are becoming wise to this.

The contemporary interpretation of the ancestral diet has seen an explosion of popularity in the mainstream over the last decade, manifesting itself as the "paleo diet," "the zone diet," "the caveman diet," "the hunter-gatherer diet," "the warrior diet," "primal living," "evolutionary eating," and more. Along with a growing number of scientists, some of the people behind these diets and lifestyles have become the thought leaders of the ancestral health movement. 'Ancestral' is an academic word that fully captures the scope of human evolution (including both the Paleolithic and the Neolithic rise of civilization), and is a word that has already been offered as an umbrella term for the overall movement to recognize the importance of an evolutionary perspective, most notably by the Ancestral Health Society, a foundation whose goal is to foster collaboration among scientists, health professionals, and laypersons who study and communicate about health from an evolutionary perspective.

Behind the greater ancestral health movement are experts and laypersons representing a diverse set of fields and expertise. They are devoted to spreading ideas about health, evolution, food, and lifestyle. Many of these individuals are formally trained at advanced levels. They are biochemists, neurobiologists, medical doctors, researchers, psychologists, nutritionists, dieticians, as well as professionals outside the realm of health and medicine, such as economists and journalists. (For a list of websites and books by these and others, see Appendix A: Resources.)

Like any discipline, there is some level of disagreement on all kinds of things, from food to history to evolution to exercise to organization to you-name-it. But the many burgeoning ideologies are more alike than different, because they share a unifying concept: that evolution can improve lives by shedding light on human nature. Rather than simply offering my own personal view of the ancestral health diet debate, I intend to portray the spectrum of ideology to some degree and to give a general representation of common interpretations of the ancestral diet, based on the diverse array of ideologies circulating within the world of ancestral health — our best place to look in order to answer the far-reaching question, *what is the natural human diet?*

A Diet Defined by the Wild, Interpreted by the Experts

Without further ado, let's dive right into the ancestral diet as it translates to the world today, as commonly recommended by experts and thought leaders in the field. This diet includes primarily vegetables, seafood, eggs, meat, and roots/tubers/starchy veggies, and it highlights the importance of obtaining high-quality, toxin-free food (wild, grass-finished, grass-fed, organic, biodynamic, local). The diet also includes varying degrees of fruits, organ meats, nuts, and seeds.

The big picture is to eat real food as close as possible to how it would be available in the wild, but also to include modern foods that are clearly beneficial. This generally means restricting sugar, vegetable oils, grains, legumes, and dairy, and also avoiding pesticides, herbicides, preservatives, industrial meats, industrial produce, canned goods, and processed foods. There are, however, some exceptions, which we'll cover later.

A lot of these things are a no-brainer, but actually avoiding 'Neolithic' foods like sugar and vegetable oils can be a struggle. Sugar can find its way into nearly everything we eat: sauces, condiments, restaurant dishes, health drinks, and juices. So right away, it should be clear to anyone on the Standard American Diet (SAD) that their usual shopping practices will have to change. As will their definition of food. And their connection to food.

An easy rule of thumb for following the diet easily is to stick to the core essentials (organic vegetables, pastured meats, and roots/tubers/starchy veggies) and treat all other foods as potentially suboptimal or even toxic. I've included a few sample meal plans for the Optimal Eater, the Average Joe, and the Starving Musician, all based on budget (see Appendix B).

One of the universal ideas in the ancestral health world is the disdain for the Low-Fat Diet Craze. Although understanding the biochemistry of dietary fat and its interaction with the human body can be bewildering, a few ancestral biochemists and journalists have demonstrated that it's not as simple as low-fat, but it is as simple as 'real food'. Thankfully, there are two takeaway messages about fat that are just as simple, and can be easily employed.

Fat Lesson #1: don't be scared of saturated fat.[116] In fact, cook with it preferentially and in only its purest forms, things like butter from the milk of grass-fed cows, coconut oil, and ghee, all of which can be found in health food stores. The stable chemical structure of saturated fat makes it less likely to oxidize (burn) than other cooking oils and fats. Oxidation is worth avoiding because it may cause heart disease.[117] Additionally, today's experts no longer

---

[116] Taubes, Gary. *Good Calories, Bad Calories.* Knopf, 2007.

[117] Staprans et al (2005). The role of dietary oxidized cholesterol and oxidized fatty acids in the

vilify fat:

> Based on modern advances in nutritional science, including prospective cohort studies of disease outcomes and randomized controlled trials of disease outcomes, it is now widely acknowledged that the proportion of calories from total fat has no appreciable effect on risk of CHD or cancers. Decades ago, it would have been seen as heresy to make such a statement. However, advances in nutritional science now render this conclusion quite obvious, as affirmed by recent expert reports from both the World Health Organization and the World Cancer Research Fund...
>
> Although the paradigm that saturated fat is a major cause of CHD has become entrenched in the public and scientific consciousness over decades, modern nutritional evidence simply does not support a major effect of saturated fat on CHD risk. [118]

Fat has been a major source of dietary calories for humans for hundreds of thousands of years (it's present in animal tissues)[119] — indeed, humans have eaten animals for millions of years. Hunter-gatherers today eat plenty of saturated fat in animal foods — about as much as Westerners do — yet don't get cardiovascular disease.[120] Natural food sources, including animal foods, are by definition adaptive. It makes zero evolutionary sense that they would cause disease. Would eating mice give snakes heart disease? Evolution calls out the absurdity of that question. Studies linking meat to disease are mixed. Some

---

development of atherosclerosis. *Molecular Nutrition and Food Research* 49(11):1075-82.

[118] Mozaffarian, D (2011). The Great Fat Debate: Taking the Focus Off of Saturated Fat. *Journal of the American Dietetic Association* 111 (5): 665-666.

[119] Ben-Dor et al (2011). Man the Fat Hunter: the demise of homo erectus and the emergence of a new hominin lineage in the middle Pleistocene (ca. 400 kyr) Levant. *PLoS ONE* 6(12): e28689.

[120] Cordain et al (2002). The paradoxical nature of hunter-gatherer diets: meat-based, yet non-atherogenic. *European Journal of Clinical Nutrition* 56 (1): S42-52.

show no relationship at all with diseases like heart disease, stroke, and diabetes.[121]

Dietary saturated fat is a clean source of energy. After all, our own bodies have saturated fat stores in them; we are quite literally fat-burning machines. Dietary saturated fat helps us uptake fat-soluble vitamins and minerals. And it can have a soothing effect on a potentially irritated gut-tract, which is highly sensitive to food toxins and a vital barrier between our bloodstream and the contents of our intestines.

Fat Lesson #2: avoid omega-6. This is a type of unsaturated fatty acid that sneaks its way into many Neolithic foods. We are evolved to consume low levels of this fat due to its scarcity in nature, but it is common today in oils and foodstuffs, promoting inflammation by throwing off the omega 3:6 ratio.[122] It's popularly known today that eating omega-3's is a good idea, but science has shown that it's the omega 3:6 ratio that really counts toward inflammation. Eating less omega-6, therefore, restores balance to the ratio without the need of supplementing omega-3, a relatively unstable fatty acid prone to oxidation and rancidity.[123] (Although, getting omega-3s in the diet via fish and grass-fed meats is a good idea.) An updated 2012 meta-analysis of the Sydney Diet Heart Study illuminates the inevitable damage of omega-6 to human health:

>...substituting dietary linoleic acid [an omega-6 polyunsaturated fat] in place of saturated fats increased the rates of death from all causes, coronary heart disease, and cardiovascular disease.[124]

---

[121] Micha, Wallace, and Mozaffarian (2010). Red and processed meat consumption and risk of incident coronary heart disease, stroke, and diabetes: a review and meta-analysis. *Circulation* 121 (21): 2271-2283.

[122] Simopoulos, A.P. (2002). The importance of the ratio of omega-6/omega-3 fatty acids. *Biomedicine and Pharmacotherapy* 56(8): 365-379.

[123] Eades and Eades. *Protein Power Lifeplan.* Grand Central, 2001. Also discussed in blog post: "Oxidized fish oil." Retrieved from http://www.proteinpower.com/drmike/uncategorized/oxidized-fish-oil/

[124] Ramsden et al (2013). Use of dietary linoleic acid for secondary prevention of coronary heart disease and death: evaluation of recovered data from Sydney Diet Heart Study and updated meta-

With an out-of-scale inflammatory response, our bodies are unable to heal effectively. Also, symptoms will worsen for anyone with an inflammatory condition, which includes many diseases, from acne to eczema to allergies to irritable bowel syndrome.

Avoiding omega-6 is a cinch if you're following an ancestral diet, because omega-6 exists predominantly in vegetable and seed cooking oils and industrially-raised meats. Vegetable oil is not made from vegetables, and seeds naturally contain high amounts of omega-6 when concentrated into oil. Industrially-raised animals are a slew of toxins, from omega-6 to antibiotics to hormones to bacterial pathogens, while a healthy grass-fed or pastured farm animal will have virtually none of the toxins found in industrially-raised animals. This is due to the animal's diet and health. In a feedlot, cows are fed grains to fatten them up, but grains are not what cows evolved to eat. The grain destroys the cow's natural fermentative digestion system. As a consequence, they become fat, sick, and nearly dead. Unhealthy cows living in unnaturally close and unsanitary quarters need antibiotics in order to stem the spread of disease, which furthers the cow's deteriorating health up to the point of slaughter. Contrast this with a naturally raised cow on a small local farm that eats grass and roams free, as cows evolved to live. Industrially-raised animals are unhealthy, unhappy, and obese until finally slaughtered; cows on real farms are healthy, happy, and more delicious to boot! As the legendary chef Julia Child recommends, "Learn where the meat comes from." That's the route to enjoying better-tasting food.

Plants vs. Animals

Much of the debate surrounding the constitution of the ancestral diet is in regard to macronutrient proportions (fat, carb, and protein ratios) and the emphasis on food categories (plants vs. animals). One end of ancestral diet advice is in the realm of high-fat/low-carb eating, which emphasizes healthy fats, animal proteins, and vegetables instead of starches, grains, and fruits. This advice has been especially resonant for people looking to curb obesity, diabetes, and gut issues. While the importance of animal consumption to human evolution is well supported,[125][126][127] our gut physiology is strikingly similar to other primates,[128] suggesting that our modern physiology stems from our hominid ancestors who ate leaves and fruit and go back over 25 million years.

On the other end of the spectrum is an emphasis on plants over animal foods. This eating pattern sticks to starchy veggies, roots, tubers, healthy oils, and fruit in order to obtain calories. A small amount of animal products is encouraged, preferring fish and pastured eggs above other types of meat. This also emphasizes eating a significant amount of vegetables, and allows some well-prepared beans and some "safe" whole grains, like rice, sorghum, buckwheat, and tapioca. Some within this realm extend the logic of evolution from ~3.4 million years of plant and animal consumption, to the over 25 million years of hominids that consumed a plant-based[129] diet.[130]

The middle road is perhaps the one best representative of a moderated ancestral diet. It includes a balance of carbs, proteins, and fats. It makes sense for healthy folks to include carbs in the diet so that the body doesn't need to manufacture glucose from other molecules, which is an inefficient process, in turn affecting energy levels.[131] Good amounts of healthy fats are included, although lower than other high-fat adherents, and about half to most of the

---

[125] Mann, Neil (2007). Meat in the human diet: an anthropological perspective. *Nutrition and Dietetics* 64: S102-S107.

[126] Stanford and Bunn. *Meat-eating and Human Evolution.* Oxford University Press, 2001.

[127] Crawford et al (1999). Evidence for the unique function of docosahexaenoic acid (DHA) during the evolution of the modern hominid brain. *Lipids* S39–S47.

[128] Milton and Demment (1998). Digestive and passage kinetics of chimpanzees fed high and low fiber diets and comparison with human data. *Journal of Nutrition* 118:1.

[129] Kay RF (1977). Diet of early Miocene hominoids. *Nature* 268: 628–30.

[130] Milton, Katharine (2000). Hunter-gatherer diets: a different perspective. *American Journal of Clinical Nutrition* 71(3): 665-667.

[131] Jaminet and Jaminet. *Perfect Health Diet.* YinYang Press, 2010.

volume of food is in the form of vegetables. To some degree, all ancestral diet adherents have meals that waver across the spectrum of macronutrient proportion on a meal-to-meal basis.

Perhaps the most interesting analysis of macronutrient proportions comes from the Jaminets' *Perfect Health Diet*, which points to human milk production and human body composition as indicators of optimal macronutrient proportions. Human milk, by calories, contains 39% carbs, 54% fat, and 7% protein.[132] The Jaminets write, "We can trust that evolution has designed milk to provide infants with optimal ratios." That evolutionary logic is further refined by the composition of the adult human body, which contains 74% fat and 26% protein by calories.[133] With carbs added for the brain at 20%, that leaves an approximate proportion of 20% carbs, 60% fat, and 20% protein, again perhaps hinting at an optimal ratio.[134] This eat-what-your-body-needs approach may lessen the amount of work the body must do in converting nutrients. While the logic behind this may be hard to grasp, these are some of the best clues we have as to optimal proportions of macronutrients.

The emphasis on plants vs. animals will depend largely on the individual's goals. Are you eating to enjoy your food? Are you eating to cut fat? Are you eating to build muscle? Do you consider meat-eating ethical? These and other considerations must be made in order for each individual to strike their own balance with regard to emphasizing plants vs. animals. Many people believe the style of the ancestral diet doesn't matter as much as the guiding principle: just eat real food.

The Evolutionary Logic Behind Real Food

The important takeaway message — eat real food — is resonant for many

---

[132] George and DeFrancesca. Human milk in comparison to cow milk. In: Lebenthals, ed. Texbook of Gastroenterology and Nutrition. New York: Raven Press, 1989: 239-261.

[133] Wang et al (1992). The five-level model: a new approach for organizing body-composition research. *American Journal of Clinical Nutrition* 56 (1): 19-28.

[134] Jaminet and Jaminet. *Perfect Health Diet.* YinYang Press, 2010.

inside and outside the world of ancestral health.[135] For many ancestral health experts, other considerations are of secondary importance. Lowering disease-risk and achieving health benefits stems almost entirely from simply choosing real food. Indeed, this may be the most important aspect of dietary health.

I have been ecstatic to see the popularization of real food over the last decade by prominent authors like Michael Pollan and by commercial successes like Whole Foods. But real food can only be understood in evolutionary terms, because it was the foods available in the wild that are truly 'natural' to the human diet. Katherine Milton, anthropologist at the University of California, Berkeley has emphasized choosing foods that resemble those throughout time and as available in the wild.[136] Evolution helps us to see that whole foods aren't good for us because they are natural, nor because they are 'real' — they are good for us because *Homo sapiens sapiens* evolved to eat foods available in the wild. This is the underlying logical justification for eating natural foods, important because it sidesteps the naturalistic fallacy committed by the prevailing dietary ethos of our time.

Many people in the world of ancestral health do not concern themselves with macronutrient proportions or calorie counting, instead focusing on real food in order to achieve better health. The Industrial Revolution is the most potent historical event that changed the human diet, introducing foods like processed grains (rather than cultivated grains) and refined sugar, which significantly increased caloric intake and glycemic load while decreasing satiety and nutrition — both have been clearly linked to the development of chronic Western diseases.[137] Simply choosing real food helps us to ignore all of the invented human foods that have been linked to disease. Thus, defining real food in the light of evolution and choosing real food as a baseline for the diet is a surprisingly simple and elegant solution to an infinitely complex and

---

[135] Pollan, Michael. *In Defense of Food: an Eater's Manifesto.* Penguin, 2009.

[136] Milton, Katherine (2002). Hunter-gatherer diets: wild foods signal relief from diseases of affluence. In Ungar and Teaford (Eds.). *Human Diet: its Origin and Evolution.*

[137] Elton and Higgins. "Environment, Adaptation, and Evolutionary Medicine." *Evolution and Medicine: Current Applications, Future Prospects.* Boca Raton: CRC Press, 2008.

highly politicized problem.

Appetite and Satiety

Appetite and satiety are often overlooked aspects of the health debate. However, there are many lifestyle factors that influence the increase and decrease in appetite. Exercise has long been considered a potent appetite stimulant and intensifier due to increased caloric requirements, but it also paradoxically increases satiety at a fixed meal.[138] Sleep also greatly affects appetite. Sleep deprivation can increase appetite by decreasing leptin levels in the body (leptin is a hormone that regulates energy intake and expenditure) and increasing ghrelin (a hunger-stimulating hormone), leading not only to increased appetite, but also increased desire for high-calorie foods.[139] Exercise and sleep research confirms commonly held notions that they are beneficial to health by controlling appetite.

Fasting is also an important topic related to diet, health, and nutrition. From an evolutionary perspective, our ancestors fasted regularly simply out of necessity. Food was scarce and available inconsistently, so they likely bore the brunt of short periods of famine. Many recent studies confirm that fasting can be beneficial to the health of the modern human, although females may not see some of its benefits.[140] [141] Fasting is a way of cutting calories, which can incite weight loss and may increase lifespan. Fasting also incites a period of cellular self-eating that paradoxically instigates repair, healing, and regulation

---

[138] King et al (2008). Dual-process action of exercise on appetite control. *American Journal of Clinical Nutrition* 90(4): 921-927.

[139] Spiegel et al (2004). Sleep curtailment in healthy young men associated with decreased leptin levels, elevated ghrelin levels, and increased hunger and appetite. *Annals of Internal Medicine* 141(11):846-850.

[140] Heilbronn et al (2005). Glucose tolerance and skeletal muscle gene expression in response to alternate day fasting. *Obesity Research* 13 (3): 574-581.

[141] Heilbronn et al (2005). Alternate-day fasting in nonobese subjects: effects on body weight, body composition, and energy metabolism. *American Journal of Clinical Nutrition* 81 (1): 69-73.

in a process called autophagy.[142] Autophagic dysfunction is implicat cancer, neurodegeneration, microbial infection, aging, and heart disease.[143] Therefore, autophagy may play a role in improving human health and lengthening life span.[144] [145] Autophagy is upregulated by external stressors like starvation, suggesting that it's an important survival response.[146] Thus, its role in human evolution is a crucial one, and may be behind the health benefits of fasting. Autophagy is an evolved trait in human biological systems that can be leveraged through controlled fasting.

Fasts typically vary from skipping meals (preferably breakfast to keep the sleeping fast going) to whole 24-hour periods without food (water is allowed). More than 24-hours may lead to loss in athletic performance via breakdown of muscle tissue, so that tends to be the upper limit on the practice. Some people fast as often as daily; others as little as once a week. Also, protein-fasting has been offered as a compromise. It allows meals that do not contain animal protein or high-protein plant foods (like tofu). Restricting protein in this way may also spur autophagy and the health benefits along with it. One can optimize autophagy times easily by skipping breakfast daily. Most people find that their body will adjust to this eating pattern over time. However, fasting may be unnecessary or detrimental to highly active individuals, young people, women, athletes, and perhaps others. Seeking the advice of a health professional for one's unique situation is advisable, and self-analysis is key.

Opposite to fasting is the uncharacteristic yet highly celebrated 'cheat meal', where dieters indulge in any food their palate desires. Most diet gurus, regardless of their background, embrace the philosophy that adhering 100% to

---

[142] Yorimitsu T, Klionsky DJ (2005). Autophagy: molecular machinery for self-eating. *Cell Death and Differentiation* 12: 1542–1552.

[143] Mizushima et al (2009). Autophagy fights disease through cellular self-digestion. *Nature* 451(7182): 1069–1075.

[144] Jio and Levine (2007). Autophagy is required for dietary restriction-mediated life span extension in C. elegans. *Autophagy* 3 (6): 597–599.

[145] Hansen et al (2008). A role for autophagy in the extension of lifespan by dietary restriction in C. elegans. *PLoS Genetics* 4 (2): e42.

[146] Martinet et al (2009). Autophagy in disease. *Clinical Science* 116: 697–712.

any diet is unnecessary. Most recommend that 10-20% of meals can be allowed to be outside the realm of ancestral foods, even if they are indulgent choices like ice cream and dark chocolate. The economic model of Diminishing Marginal Utility[147] demonstrates that as one consumes more and more healthy food, there is a decline in the marginal benefit of each additional healthy food item.[148] As such, once one has consumed 80-90% of their diet in healthful food, the remaining amount of food will be of small marginal benefit. The opportunity cost (the value of the alternative) is diminished to some degree, then, when substituting the last 10-20% of healthy food with an indulgent cheat meal.

Also, there may be a psychological component to the cheat meal. Often, dieters are under a lot of stress and pressure with a new diet. When there is too much pressure to adhere to a diet plan, one may become frustrated at being unable to adhere, perhaps giving up on the diet altogether. The allowance of cheating then dissipates that pressure, ensuring that the participant is more likely to stay the course. Many argue that the degree of cheating is simply proportional to one's ambition and discipline, so finding one's own comfort zone is essential.

Lastly, about the cheat meal, I would posit a philosophical position, which is to say that the meaning of life is not perfect health. Health may very well be one of the most important goals in life, but there are experiences worth having during the short and beautiful time we have on Earth that will vie with our health goals. Whether that is the occasional dessert or getting tipsy with college buddies, there is bountiful meaning and joy, a beautiful diversity of experience, to be had in this glimmer of a lifetime. There's no wisdom in denying yourself a reasonable amount of fun while you can.

---

[147] McCulloch, James Huston (1977). The Austrian Theory of the Marginal Use and of Ordinal Marginal Utility. *Journal of Economics* 37 (3-4): 249-280.

[148] Jaminet and Jaminet. *Perfect Health Diet.* YinYang Press, 2010.

Fat Storage and Fat Burning

Or: why you should be offended by health professionals

You hear it all the time: fat storage is caused by caloric imbalance. People eat too much and don't exercise enough. In fact, this is the official definition of the cause of obesity by the National Institutes of Health and the World Health Organization. This is the answer they give for metabolic syndrome and for the overweight. It underpins their advice on cutting body fat and getting back to a healthy weight. Yet we're fatter than ever, and no one seems to be able to figure out what to do about it. As we will see, this is due to oversimplified thinking about fat accumulation. That's what got us here. I will argue that the idea of 'caloric imbalance' as a cause of fat accumulation is so obviously wrong that it's an insult to your intelligence. And yes, you should be offended.

Calories matter. That idea has been known for quite some time,[149] and confirmed over and over.[150 151 152] However, 'caloric imbalance' plays a role in accumulating fat only insofar as eating too much is a requirement of getting fat. Losing fat, they say, requires 'eating less' (a nice euphemism for starving!). Of course, this says nothing as to the *cause* or the *why* of what makes people eat too much or what turns those extra calories into fat. Imagine the conversation:

"Hey, why do people get fat?"

"Oh, that's because they eat too many calories and don't expend enough calories."

---

[149] Kinsell et al (1964). Calories do count. *Metabolism* 13 (3): 195-204.

[150] Bray et al (2012). Effect of dietary protein content on weight gain, energy expenditure, and body composition during overeating: a randomized controlled trial. *Journal of the American Medical Association* 307 (1): 47-55.

[151] Strasser et al (2007). Fat loss depends on energy deficit only, independently of the method of weight loss. *Annals of Nutrition and Metabolism* 51 (5): 428-32.

[152] Thomson et al. (2008). The effect of a hypocaloric diet with and without exercise training on body composition, cardiometabolic risk profile, and reproductive function in overweight and obese women with polycystic ovary syndrome. *The Journal of Clinical Endocrinology and Metabolism* 93 (9): 3383-90.

See how that's just a restatement of the problem, and not an answer to the question? To say that people get fat because they eat more than they expend is to say that they eat too much, which is to say absolutely nothing that we didn't already know! This is no answer, because it still hasn't addressed what *causes* the fat storage or what limits the fat burning or what leads to overeating. They might as well tell us that we eat too much and don't poop enough. Feeling offended yet?

The Calorie Hypothesis also becomes problematic as a cause of fat accumulation when you look at certain populations. In statistics, if you find a correlation between two things, then you've made an observation; if you find no correlation, then you've made a conclusion — that the two things are unrelated. Sure, there is a correlation between eating too much and being fat. However, there are a few populations that call this correlation into question.

There are scientists in the lab that have observed mice getting fat while in caloric deficit. Gary Taubes notes that they "lost 60 percent of their body fat before they died of starvation, but still had five times as much body fat as lean mice."[153] A study examining traditional societies found,

> ...average daily energy expenditure of traditional Hadza foragers was no different than that of Westerners after controlling for body size...human daily energy expenditure may be an evolved physiological trait largely independent of cultural differences.[154]

In the wild, blaming calories doesn't work. In the laboratory, the link between energy intake and expenditure is highly problematic. Could it be that biology is subject to biological laws and not mathematical laws?

The slope gets more slippery looking at obvious examples as well. Many physically demanding jobs, such as construction, see workers that gain weight despite their high levels of physical activity, which should be guarding them from fat storage by increasing their caloric needs. And, more confusingly,

---

[153] Taubes, Gary. *Good Calories, Bad Calories.* Anchor, 2008. p 366.
[154] Pontzer et al (2012). Hunter-Gatherer Energetics and Human Obesity. *PLoS ONE* 7(7): e40503.

among athletes, almost all of whom spend multiple years in caloric surplus, some become overweight but most don't. These populations call out just how ridiculous caloric imbalance is as an answer to the fat question because they demonstrate a conclusion: that the two things are unrelated. Conclusions should rightly supersede observations. It must be something else that is driving fat into our fat cells, limiting fat burning, or leading to overeating.

Fat Theories That Fit

In order to understand body fatness, we must first affirm the complexity of human biology. Then, we must move past simple correlates to fat storage (like habits, emotions, lifestyle) in order to recognize the ultimate underlying causes and bio-mechanisms. In the words of obesity researcher Stephan Guyenet:

> The brain is the main physiological control center of the body, and it communicates in both directions with almost every organ. It regulates the pulse rate of the heart, breathing rate via the diaphragm, blood pressure via the blood vessel walls and kidneys, regulates temperature by controlling sweat glands, hair follicles and capillaries in the skin, regulates various aspects of digestion, bone metabolism, glucose production by the liver, and many other functions. So it's not much of a surprise that it also controls fatty acids moving into and out of fat tissue... the brain not only controls energy intake and energy expenditure — factors that are obviously important determinants of fat mass — it also influences how much fat is moving into and out of fat tissue from the circulation by acting directly on fat cells.[155]

---

[155] Guyenet, S (2012). "What puts fat into fat cells and what takes it out?" *Whole Health Source*. [Web file] Retrieved from http://wholehealthsource.blogspot.com/2012/06/what-puts-fat-into-fat-cells-and-what.html

Considering fat storage and fat burning from an evolutionary perspective, the role of the brain makes perfect sense. Fat storage and fat burning mechanisms are evolved traits that naturally balance our weight in order to bolster survival and reproductive fitness. The brain regulates this process in healthy folks, but for the obese, this regulatory system in the brain has gone haywire.

A critical role in fat storage and fat burning is played by hormones. For decades, we've known that insulin drives glucose into fat cells, and that other hormones mobilize fat energy for burning. These hormonal mechanisms play out the actual role of fat storage and fat mobilization, driving energy into the fat cell and removing it. The important question then becomes: what influences these hormonal cascades that ultimately control fat storage and fat mobilization? Unfortunately, the entire picture is unclear, but there are a couple things we know that hint strongly toward actionable strategies.

One largely unrecognized aspect of body fatness is the fact that our hormonal systems are evolved traits. They evolved in nature according to the environment and the dictates for survival and reproduction. The implications are staggering, because they help us to see the big picture about fat. Most people see it this way: evolution teaches us that fat accumulation grants a survival advantage, storing fat during times of plenty in order to utilize it in times of scarcity. In the ancestral environment, "times of plenty" probably meant summer, when ripe fruit was bountiful, game was plentiful, and life was relatively good.

But all this may not be as simple as commonly thought. Ask yourself: is there an evolutionary advantage to promoting fat stores? Of course there is, but this is true only up to a point. Clearly, there is little evolutionary advantage to being overweight or obese, because it affects one's physical capabilities, reproductive potential, and health. And, since our ancestors maintained high levels of physical activity,[156] it is likely that those in caloric surplus came to look a lot more like modern-day athletes, the great majority of

---

[156] Cordain et al (1998). Physical activity, energy expenditure, and fitness: an evolutionary perspective. *International Journal of Sports Medicine* 19 (5): 328-335.

whom are themselves in caloric surplus. When you combine ancestral activity patterns with the fact that human ancestors did not have access to fattening Western foods, you get an interesting interpretation of natural energy storage mechanisms.

Evolution paradoxically turns the 'summer fat' idea on its head by backing the 'summer muscle' idea: humans naturally store additional muscle when in caloric surplus, as well as fat, in a homeostatic balance. Supporting this idea is the fact that muscle is itself mostly fat, and an efficient source of conversion to meet the needs of our bodies:

> Muscle, by calories, is about 74% fat and 26% protein — just right to meet the body's glucose, protein, and fat needs after conversion of some protein to glucose.[157]

Athletes and bodybuilders have long known that being in caloric surplus is *necessary* to gain muscle, which they often achieve with a calorie-dense diet. Let me repeat this: it is necessary to eat more calories than are expended, even after correcting for high levels of caloric output via exercise, in order to gain muscle. According to the World Health Organization, shouldn't bodybuilders also become obese since they spend years in caloric surplus? The math, nor the logic, check out. Even endurance athlete's muscle gains are attributable to excess calories.[158] Of course, these populations do not accumulate significant amounts of adipose tissue. Quite the riddle, except in the light of evolution.

In the coming sections, we will explore the causes of fat storage from an evolutionary perspective, and ultimately conclude that Neolithic foods and the contemporary lifestyle are at the core of what leads to the fattening of modern humans. If it is the case that natural foods do not cause body fatness, then where did all those extra calories go for our active ancestors, who undoubtedly

---

[157] Jaminet and Jaminet. *Perfect Health Diet.* YinYang Press, 2010. p 80.

[158] Stearns et al (2010). Effects of ingesting protein in combination with carbohydrate during exercise on endurance performance: a systematic review with meta-analysis. *Journal of Strength and Conditioning Research* 24 (8): 2192-2202.

had times in caloric surplus consisting of real food? You guessed it: the muscle, as well as the fat, in a naturally homeostatic balance, regulated by a complex system of comprising evolved traits that bolstered survivability and reproductive fitness.

The 'summer fat' idea is generally known as the *thrifty gene hypothesis*, which states that the environments of our ancestors selected for genes that promote fat storage in a way that was advantageous to survival and reproduction.[159] The thrifty gene hypothesis has been criticized, but its overall ideas point to some kind of genetic basis for the expression of these modern diseases. This logic is sound, especially when looking specifically at evolved traits that contribute to fat accumulation and the genetic basis of those traits. But it's the expression of those traits within the context of the Western diet that leads to disease, not necessarily within the context of calories. In understanding human well-being, it is critical to view the human evolutionary legacy within the confines of modernity and the pressures of civilization.

Insulin and Carbs

In the summer, there are more carbohydrates available in the wild via the sugars in ripening fruits. In combination with increased food supply, these carbohydrates may predict that sugar plays a role in storing body fat. Indeed, there would be a survival advantage to augment fat stores at this time. If carbohydrate availability is a reliable indicator of the summer fattening season, then carbs fit an evolutionary perspective as a signal and contributor to increased fat storage in humans. In the wild, sugars are rare and their availability is limited. In the modern world, these sugars are refined and distributed, making them more potent and available endlessly, which contributes to fat accumulation and disease. This is a prediction, but it turns out that there may be something more to this.

---

[159] Neel, JV (1962). Diabetes Mellitus: A "Thrifty" Genotype Rendered Detrimental by "Progress"? *American Journal of Human Genetics* 14 (4): 353–362.

Nutritional scientists have long known the role that insulin plays in driving glucose into fat cells. They have also long known that carbohydrates in the diet are directly tied to insulin levels. The carbs in the diet are quickly broken down into sugars in the bloodstream, where insulin is released by the pancreas to manage the sugars. What is not so commonly known is that the pancreas evolved in an environment vastly different than today's. It was not bombarded thrice daily by easily digestible carbs seen in refined sugar, juices, and processed grains and flours. Today's chronic stress on the pancreas may be a key to understanding fat accumulation from an evolutionary perspective.

In the book *Why We Get Fat,* author and *New York Times* columnist Gary Taubes addresses the important role of insulin as a bio-mechanism of fat storage and disease. In this work, he wholly rejects the calories in-calories out model of obesity, and places the blame instead on carbohydrates and the role of hormones:

> [Restricting carbohydrates] ...leads to weight loss and particularly fat loss, independent of the calories we consume from dietary protein. We know that the laws of physics have nothing to do with it.[160]

The model of caloric imbalance has been a part of nutritional dogma long enough that many consider it fact. However, Taubes, like many in the ancestral health community, deny that the body is perfectly scaled to the laws of thermodynamics. This stems back to the worldview of health institutions, which tend to look at the human body as a 'designed' system based on math. However, an evolutionary perspective highlights that the body is not a perfectly designed system at all. Instead, the human body is a collection of compromising evolved traits optimized for reproduction — not health. It's based on biology, not math. Indeed, evolution helps us to deconstruct and redefine how calories are applicable to human metabolism.

---

[160] Taubes, Gary. *Why We Get Fat: and What to Do About It.* Knopf, 2010.

The Gut-Brain Axis: a Literal Mind-Body Connection

Comedian Stephen Colbert often likes to muse that he thinks with his gut. It's an ironic statement, given that the gut houses nearly enough neurons to be its own brain. And it's a fact that has spurred many big questions: Why are there so many neurons in the gut? What is the gut's importance to health? What can we do to improve our gut health? Researchers are just beginning to understand these questions.

The gut is implicated in a diverse array of diseases, from depression to obesity, and many people believe that the gut is crucially important to overall health. The presence of neurons points to the brain, since that's another location in the body with lots of neurons. How this applies to fat storage actually starts with one of the lessons of evolution.

Among species, between species, and within species, there are thriving, ancient, and dynamic ecologies. And within those, some species have developed a symbiotic relationship with other species. They help each other out. In some examples, the symbiotic relationship is so deeply intertwined that the relationship is vital to survival. If the ecosystem that upholds that relationship is altered or destroyed — it can literally kill. This is perhaps exactly what we are seeing with obesity and immune dysfunction.

Human beings have developed a symbiotic relationship with countless species of microorganisms. They live on our skin, in our eyes, in our hair, and in our guts. In fact, you are made of more foreign cells than your own cells, because those cells belong to the microbiome, the world of microorganisms that live in and around your body.[161]

In fact, you need the microorganisms in order to survive. That's where the symbiosis comes in. In the gut, there are hundreds of health-promoting

---

[161] DOE/Lawrence Berkeley National Laboratory (2012). Scientists define the healthy human microbiome. *ScienceDaily*. Retrieved from
http://www.sciencedaily.com-/releases/2012/06/120613184040.htm

bacteria that have been identified. They help digest food and they help regulate immune function. In the obese, it's found that their gut microbiome is altered from the normal state, perhaps hinting at a causal relationship. This causal relationship has been shown in mice.[162] Given the prevalence of gut-related diseases, both mental and physical, the restoration of gut health becomes an important concept.

Evolution helps us predict that a contemporary lifestyle disturbs the natural ecosystem of the gut microbiota. We now have evidence that proves this to be the case. The culprit is the Western diet, which is laden with sugars, flours, and processed grains that alter the ecosystem that the symbiotic relationship is based on.

Probiotics, the bacteria that aid digestion and immune function, require a natural habitat to survive. Their habitat, as it has been for millions of years, is the food you eat. They need soluble fiber, like the stuff in fruits, vegetables, and tubers. Funny, because these coincide with what you'd expect given evolutionary history. Grains and legumes are, on the other hand, mostly composed of insoluble fiber, which does not provide habitat for these helpful bacteria.

At the same time, sugars and refined carbohydrate promote the growth of other unnatural microorganisms. These bad guys compete for resources with the good guys and can often cause their own problems beyond just gassiness and discomfort. However, as scary as that may be, the prescription is easy: avoid Neolithic foods.

Food Reward and Palatability

Food-related biological systems play a role in the accumulation of fat. One of the most potent influences over human behavior is the reward system of the brain. This reward system evolved to incentivize eating foods that

---

[162] Turnbaugh et al (2008). Diet-induced obesity is linked to marked but reversible alterations in the mouse distal gut microbiome. *Cell Host and Microbe* 3(4):213-223.

provided an evolutionary advantage, a system that manifested as a preference for sweet, salty, savory, and fatty foods. These taste preferences are rare in nature, so our detection systems for them are very sensitive, which explains why our palatability for them is heightened in the modern day.

Palatability is the satisfaction, or hedonic reward, derived from consuming foods and fluids. This is rooted in our need to consume them. Palatability is also a dynamic force, where foods and fluids are more palatable when deprived.

As we are just beginning to understand, behaviors surrounding food are influenced by the brain based on hormonal regulation. Food is intimately tied to our neurological reward system. We are incentivized to not only prefer rewarding foods, but to consume them whenever possible. The trouble is that the modern world has virtually unlimited availability of energy-dense, highly palatable foods. This drives behavior that would not have been possible in the ancestral environment based on availability. The discord between this reward system and modern life leads to overconsumption of energy-dense foods, which may be an important contributing factor to the development of obesity.[163] It may therefore also contribute to weight gain in normal folks, and may even play a role in obesity-related diseases. All this simply because, on a neurobiological level, we are designed by nature to seek out rewarding foods.

Evolution and Gender: Feminist Perspectives on Fat

Men and women share many biological features, but many are also distinct. One common theme in the evolution of any life form is its ability to adapt to the challenges of its environment. The greater the challenge, the more impressive the adaptation. From the long neck of the giraffe to the sticky pads of the salamander's feet, the challenges of nature have spurred some remarkable adaptations.

---

[163] Guyenet and Schwartz (2012). Clinical review: Regulation of food intake, energy balance, and body fat mass: implications for the pathogenesis and treatment of obesity. *Journal of Clinical Endocrinology and Metabolism* 97 (3): 745-755.

One potent evolved trait — and one that is unique to females — is the ability to give life. Of course, I'm talking about pregnancy. Pregnàncy is one way that nature has challenged our female ancestors. With the increased survival pressure of pregnancy, women have evolved traits that are distinct from their male counterparts.

Much to the chagrin of today's fashionistas, the human female evolved the ability to promote fat stores more readily than males. This is evident due to gender differences in the homeostatic set point for body fat, as well as in food preferences.

Women naturally maintain a higher body fat percentage than men, and are more likely to store it in their lower extremities; men are more likely to store fat on the abdomen.[164] Essential body fat composition is typically 3-5% in men and 8-12% in women.[165] This difference is due to the demands of carrying and raising children. In the ancestral environment, women needed that extra fat as stored energy in order to bolster survival for themselves and their offspring. Female biology has adapted to the added survival pressure of pregnancy.

Women love their sweets, surely. Is that also attributable to evolution? In fact, women prefer sweets, fruits, and vegetables more than men do.[166] They exhibit a taste preference for sweets in their day-to-day lives,[167] according to their menstrual cycle,[168] and over the course of their pregnancy.[169] Because there was an evolutionary advantage in the ancestral environment to storing

---

[164] Power and Schulkin (2008). Sex differences in fat storage, fat metabolism, and health risks from obesity: possible evolutionary origins. *British Journal of Nutrition* 99 (5): 931-940.

[165] Fahey, Insel, and Roth. "Body Composition". *Fit & Well: Core Concepts and Labs in Physical Fitness and Wellness*. McGraw-Hill, 2010.

[166] Caine-Bish and Scheule (2009). Gender differences in taste preferences in school-aged children and adolescents. *Journal of School Health* 29 (11).

[167] Logue and Smith (1986). Predictors of food preferences in adult humans. *Appetite* 7 (2): 109-125.

[168] Bowen and Grundberg (1990). Variation in food preference and consumption across the menstrual cycle. *Physiology and Behavior* 47 (2): 287-291.

[169] Bowen, Deborah (1992). Taste and food preference changes across the course of pregnancy. *Appetite* 19 (3): 233-242.

more fat as a woman, then it is predictable that female biological mechanisms would support behaviors and choices that led to fat accumulation. In this case, the fact that women love sweets more than their male counterparts may simply be an evolved trait that helps them survive, attract mates, and reproduce.

(This observation also points to the wisdom of our bodies telling us that sweets, which are carbs, are more fattening. This is, of course, why women prefer sweets more than men do — precisely *because* they make us fat. Stack this on the pile of evidence that demonstrates the role of carbohydrates in fat storage and obesity-related diseases.)

The modern world makes fat loss doubly hard for women due to the competing ideals of contemporary femininity. First, we know that perceptions of female beauty change over time according to culture. It just so happens that today, the female standard of beauty is one where skinniness is the gold standard. Books like *Skinny Bitch* fly off the shelves. Our celebrities, advertisements, and models trend toward this ideal with few exceptions.

Yet in strict evolutionary terms, skinniness is not ideal. Not for fertility, where 'plump' might be a better word. Not for attraction, where 'curvy' might be a better word. And not for utility, where 'muscular' might be a better word. All of these would detract from one's skinniness, yet skinniness remains the most popular health goal among women. This cultural phenomenon may very well be here to stay for some time. So be it.

There's nothing wrong with being skinny or wanting to be skinny. If you find yourself among those who cave to societal pressure, guess what? You're human. It's only natural to care what others think about you. We are social animals, after all. It's certainly possible to be skinny and healthy at the same time. Some women are naturally skinny and that's great.

But, as a culture, we should be careful about generally classifying any ideal body type, even skinniness. Women who struggle with weight may take things too far. They may pursue skinniness with misguided information that leads to malnourishment or detracts from their overall health. Indeed skinniness often becomes the central health goal of many women, spurring them to drastically cut calories (also known as starving) or take up marathoning (and probably overtraining) — actions that in reality will directly vie with their goal of being skinny.

I would propose an evolution-friendly alternative to the *Skinny Bitch* — something more like the *Curvy Diva* — but where are those books? A Curvy Diva would have heightened fertility levels.[170] She would be the most attractive.[171] Her modest muscle mass would slow the aging process.[172] She would be more capable in day-to-day physical activities. She would be at lower disease risk.[173] She would be free from artificial standards of body image, defining her own ideals of beauty and health according to the laws of nature. Above all, she would be gleaming with energy and vitality and would have properly laid down the foundation for a resilient mental, emotional, and spiritual self.

The irony is that feminine behavioral norms and physical ideals actually detract from the individual goals of women. Since skinniness has become a prized trait in our culture, women often eat less than they require at fixed meals in order to achieve that goal. However, this may become a cycle that works directly against the goal of skinniness.

Eating less risks increasing one's appetite, which inevitably leads to increased snacking. Snacks are almost always unhealthy. This is because when cravings are ramped up, we grab whatever is quickly satisfying, like cookies, crackers, chips, etc. — all of which contribute to overeating.[174] Additionally, if one is eating less food, then they are also eating fewer nutrients, which may

---

[170] Frisch, Rose. *Female Fertility and the Body Fat Connection.* Chicago: University of Chicago Press, 2002.

[171] Dixson et al (2010). Male preferences for female waist-to-hip ratio and body mass index in the highlands of Papua New Guinea. *American Journal of Physical Anthropology* [PDF web file] Retrieved from http://www.pngibr.org/publications/pdf/2010-Dixson-et-al.pdf.

[172] Sreekumaran Nair, K. (2005). Aging muscle. *American Journal of Clinical Nutrition* 81 (5): 953-963.

[173] Cashdan, E. (2008). Waist-to-hip ratio across cultures: trade-offs between androgen- and estrogen-dependent traits. *Current Anthropology* 49 (6): 1099-1107.

[174] Graaf, C. (2006). Effects of snacks on energy intake: an evolutionary perspective. *Appetite* 47 (1): 18-23.

lead to malnourishment. In this way, portion size at fixed meals represents one important way that culturally-influenced behavior exacerbates biological nature, only furthering the woman from her goal of skinniness. Perhaps it is poetic justice that dieting women will inevitably cave to the power of their own hunger hormones.

The Evolution of Satiety

The transition to meat-eating was one of the most important trends in human evolution, because the energy-dense animal foods that our ancestors enjoyed allowed our brains to grow. It led to nomadic behavior, spreading our species over the globe in search of food. As it turned out, there was food available almost everywhere we looked. However, the energy density of animal food meant that we needed a lot less of it. As a result, our bodies evolved 'satiety hormones' that told us when we had enough, signaling fullness during and after a meal.

The satiety hormones include leptin, ghrelin, orexin, cholecystokinin, neuropeptide Y, and agouti-related peptide. In the ancestral environment, the only types of macronutrients that required fullness, due to their energy content and abundance, were the ones in animal foods: fat and protein. The result is the evolved mechanisms of satiety that signal that we've had enough of these. These foods could easily be overindulged in, which would lead to negative outcomes. Our bodies needed satiety hormones in order avoid these negative outcomes.[175]

Carbohydrate, however, is not as potent at making us feel full. Carbs are connected to the release of putative satiety hormones, including glucagon-like peptide-1 and amylin.[176] Why would evolution guide our bodies to trigger greater fullness for fat and protein than carbs? The answer is evolutionary

[175] Meller, William. *Evolution Rx*. New York: Penguin, 2009. pp. 9.

[176] Feinle, O'Donovan, and Horowitz (2008). Carbohydrate and satiety. *Nutrition Reviews* 60 (6): 155-169.

pressure. When hunters took down a big game animal, there was ample food — one could eat themselves into oblivion if they so desired. Thus, there was pressure to evolve a trait for fullness. However, there is no carbohydrate equivalent to this in the ancestral environment. In fact, carbs were relatively rare in the ancestral environment, so there was little pressure to evolve biochemical mechanisms that limited their consumption.

There were fair amounts of slowly-digested carbs available year-round in tubers and starchy veggies, as well as in fruit in the summer. But the time and energy required to procure these foods allowed for their swift digestion without the risk of overdoing it. The ancestral environment did not favor fullness in these scenarios due to their limited availability and their biological necessity for fat storage. Also, fruits in the ancestral environment were nothing like the sugary sweet fruits today that farmers have selectively bred for thousands of years. Instead, fruits in the ancestral environment were low in sugar — something more like today's crabapple. In this environment, our biological pathways concerning carb metabolism evolved to handle low amounts of sugars. This illuminates how today's high-sugar environment overwhelms our bodies, leading to disease.

Fat accumulation, or body fatness, is ultimately a result of the interaction of food with our evolved traits. We get hungry, we get full. We store energy, we burn energy. These traits were naturally homeostatic in the ancestral environment. They achieved a balance according to evolutionary pressure. But today, our lives are out of line with these traits. We now have an endless supply of sugars, quickly-digested carbs, and calories; yet we have no appetite-controlling bio-mechanisms. Thankfully, understanding fat accumulation from an evolutionary perspective can help us reach our goals.

Strategies in Dieting

Eat real food, in evolutionary terms. Breathe clean air, drink pure water, preferably from a spring. Eat mostly vegetables by volume, as diverse an array as possible, but according to your preferences. Include some healthy fats at most meals. Protein and carb intake should be scaled to the type and intensity of physical activity; muscle-building needs more protein, endurance more carbs, and high amounts of carbs are only helpful following intense exercise. It's important to eat enough food to curb the appetite, which will prevent snacking on junk food. Those looking to cut body fat should keep an eye on limiting high-calorie foods (fats, and especially carbs). People with abdominal issues may not do well on vegetables. Otherwise, for healthy folks, eat to enjoy your meals.

Body fat has mostly to do with diet. Musculature and bone structure have mostly to do with movement. Don't commit the fallacy of working out intensely to lose fat. If you want wider shoulders, you may need to lift heavy and eat big, as Arnold Schwarzenegger recommends. Fat loss and muscle gain are both physiological adaptations, so train and eat appropriately.

Fast intermittently according to your ambition for health and longevity. Fasting is a great fat loss strategy and autophagy is an evolved trait worth exploiting, because it may lead to improved health and a longer life. Skipping breakfast is the most popular form of fasting, but experiment with what works for you. Daily to once-per-week are typical fasting frequencies. Athletes, young folks, and women may do just fine, or even better, without fasting at all.

Proactively maintain gut health. Perhaps the most important aspect of dietary health is the regulation of the system that separates nutrients from toxins entering our bodies. Therefore, it is important to avoid toxic food that will adversely affect gut health, which is pretty much anything 'Neolithic', but especially alcohol, sugar, and grains (wheat, most notably). You can promote gut health by eating fermented foods and supplementing with probiotics. Be sure to include starchy vegetables with probiotics in order to create a habitat for the bacteria, and to eat plenty of vegetables.

So what about cooking?

Where does cooking fit into the evolutionary paradigm? According to anthropologist Richard Wrangham, human ancestors probably began controlling fire about 2 million years ago, which sparked a dramatic leap in human evolution.[177] Fire led to cooking, which in turn led to more efficient digestion and energy extraction from food. It also provided warmth and protection, ultimately setting the stage for a major shift in human social formation. In other words, fire was a big deal. And so was cooking. So what does that mean for us today?

Wrapping our heads around cooking strategies can seem to be a challenge, but really this circulates around three issues: the effect of cooking on nutrient bioavailability, the effect of cooking on nutrient loss, and the effect of cooking on toxin formation. All of these things depend on cooking method, whether it's baked, fried, grilled, boiled, or whatever.

When the molecules in food undergo cooking, they see vast changes. In most food, nutrients will become more digestible, leading to increased nutrient delivery. This is especially true for common-sense items that required cooking for palatability, foods like meats, tubers, and fibrous vegetables. The opposite is true for delicate items on the other end of the spectrum. Cooking delicate foods tends to decrease the bioavailability of nutrients. (Think of how quickly spinach wilts in the frying pan.)

Some cooking methods are more efficient at preserving nutrients than others. The best choices for nutrient preservation are slow cooking, steaming, and boiling (as long you consume the broth, which

---

[177] Wrangham, Richard. *Catching Fire: How Cooking Made Us Human.* Basic, 2010.

is where many nutrients go once boiled — this is how broth is made!). Baking and pressure cooking are also great choices. It's best to avoid deep frying and grilling.

Some cooking methods actually create toxins in otherwise healthy food. Most notably, grilling is the culprit, but so are any cooking methods that lead to burning. In fact, all high-temperature cooking methods are suspect. Grilling creates two potentially cancer-causing agents: polycyclic aromatic hydrocarbons and heterocyclic amines. The hydrocarbons form from burned fat drippings and then rise up in the smoke, ultimately landing on the meat. Heterocyclic amines are created by the high temperature cooking of meat.

A good rule of thumb is to cook slowly on low temperature, using liquids whenever possible.

The Lost Foods of our Ancestors

Many foods which were common to our ancestor's diets are now uncommon in the modern diet. These include things like bone marrow, bark, sea vegetables, shellfish, insects, and organ meats. Bone marrow is a calorically-dense[178] nutritional powerhouse, providing calcium, gelatin, and whatever else (nutritional analysis on marrow is not yet performed). The Algonquin Indians of the Adirondacks derive their name from eating bark; these "tree eaters" supplemented their diet with bark in times of scarcity. Many bark-based supplements today come in bottle-form. Seaweed is a rare source of dietary iodine, which is so rare many countries require it in table salt in order to curb malnutrition in the public. Shellfish are packed with minerals. Many eat them today, but probably not as often as our coastal-dwelling ancestors did. Insects are considered to be the most sustainable source

---

[178] Cordain et al (2002).Fatty acid analysis of wild ruminant tissues: evolutionary implications for reducing diet-related chronic disease. *European Journal of Clinical Nutrition* 56(3):181-9.

of protein on the planet thanks to their enormous biomass, of which there are about 2,000 edible species. A handful of new companies have been founded to provide protein bars based on this ancient food source. Organ meats are by far the most nutrient-dense category of food across the entire spectrum of nutrition, yet many do not take advantage of liver, heart, kidneys, skin, brains, tripe, etc. All of these lost foods are a testament to how far removed humans are from nature. Many may be glad to be removed from some of these admittedly bizarre foods, but it goes to show that understanding evolution helps us to understand the current state (and future) of nutrition.

"You may reason that we have [brains] to perceive the world and to think, and that's completely wrong...We have a brain for one reason and one reason only — and that's to produce adaptable and complex movements...There can be no evolutionary advantage to laying down memories of childhood or perceiving the color of a rose if it doesn't affect how you are going to move later in life."

Daniel Wolpert

Cambridge neuroscientist

CHAPTER 4

EXPLORING THE BENEFITS OF NATURAL MOVEMENT

Throughout evolutionary history, our ancestors were forced to move as a matter of survival. Even painting an elementary picture of how they lived helps us understand how they moved. They hunted big game animals. They walked and ran long distances. They built shelter. They danced. They squatted. Thankfully, through the fields of anthropology and evolutionary biology, we now have a much clearer view about what life was like for our hunter-gatherer ancestors, and what that means for us today.

We know that physical fitness was an evolutionary given. Our ancestors were highly athletic by modern standards. By examining ancient skeletal remains, researchers have found that both women and men were well-muscled and tall relative to today.[179] They were capable of working and playing for hours, running long distances, and achieving great accuracy with weapons and tools, even well into middle age. The types of movements they performed helped to shape our bodies into what they are today.

---

[179] Ruff, C.B. (2005). Mechanical determinants of bone form: insights from skeletal remains. *Journal of Musculoskeletal and Neuronal Interactions* 5 (3): 202-212.

'Natural movement' is the concept that defines the primal human movements as we evolved in nature. The movements include walking, running, squatting, swimming, climbing, fighting, dancing, crawling, jumping, balancing, throwing, and lifting — all movements that retain precedence during the millions of years of human evolution. Indeed, these attributes were vital to our ancestors. As you may have already guessed, natural movement is at the heart of nearly any good fitness professional's philosophy.

Surprisingly, this idea is nothing new. It was first popularized in the 1800s by Georges Hebert, a French physical educator, theorist, and instructor, who had seen the impressive physicalities of the indigenous people of Africa during his travels. Back in France, he developed a system of physical fitness that he termed 'Natural Method'. It incorporated all of the movements listed above but attributed none of them to the tenets of evolution.

Think about today's mainstream Globo-Gym. It's full of treadmills, ellipticals, and stairmasters. These emphasize cardio. On the other end of the gym is usually a collection of weight sets, mostly consisting of dumbbells. The movements are simple, repetitive, and isolated. These movements are great for bodybuilding and safe for regular customers, but they do not deliver the athletic results that a natural movement program would because they do not recognize the complexity of human anatomy or even the role of the human body. They ignore the truth of how we came to move as a species and what it even means to move in the first place.

The Brain's Basic Purpose

Evolution teaches us that movement is the fundamental role of the brain. When life on Earth was in its simplest form, it needed a beginning organ to produce adaptable, complex movements. The brain filled this role and plays it still. It was upon this foundational evolutionary trait that the rest of the brain's architecture was built: logic, emotion, consciousness. The important question to ask is, how can this understanding help us recharacterize movement?

In the book *Spark: the Revolutionary New Science of Exercise and the Brain,* John J. Ratey tells a fascinating story about students in Naperville, Illinois. With the guidance of Phil Lawler, a revolutionary physical education director, students saw improvements in overall school performance simply by implementing a new PE program. Instead of grading on performance and skill, he emphasized effort and personal goals, giving good grades to those who demonstrated with a heart rate monitor that they were working to stay within their target heart rate zone. The result: more exercise. Ratey, an MD and professor at Harvard Medical School, attributes the student's academic excellence to the new PE program, explaining that the brain evolved to move the body, thus forever interweaving movement and brain function. This guides us to a profound truth: that movement makes us smarter. Can mastering movement help even more?

Athleticism is a State of Nature

So, what is athleticism? Many people debate this topic passionately. It may be one of the most misunderstood topics in physical fitness and sports theory. There are those who define the athlete broadly as simply someone who is active and capable of the demands of physical activity. Fitness professionals all seem to have their own particular version of what constitutes true athleticism, but the central ideas are the same. People who are athletic seem to always be defined against someone who is fit. Fitness, in this way, is defined as someone's physical capacity — for example, how far or how long someone can run.

The defining characteristic of athleticism, on the other hand, is adaptability, the brain's ability to control the body to produce optimal movement. A fit person trains the body; an athlete trains the mind. As a foundation, athletes possess fitness (strength, cardiovascular capacity) but also mastery of the mind-body connection: balance, posture, speed, power, agility, reaction time, visual feedback, foot work, hand-eye coordination, etc. The missing link is the addition of split-second decision-making, the ability to coordinate complexity to accomplish movement. It is an idea that brings the concept of movement full circle. Our brains are what really gauge human movement, so it is our brains that should fully define it. Athleticism, in this way, is the mastery of movement. These are the elements of physicality that lend to one's athletic prowess, their effectiveness in whatever field of sport or activity.

You're not going to the Super Bowl, so why is this relevant? Some people will be interested in developing athleticism even if not competitive athletes. Athletic training is the most effective route to fitness. Athletic training is smarter, more functional, and can be performed safely. It's literally the difference between training the mind for movement versus training the body for fitness. Its methodology can be tapered to suit individual goals. There is certainly a degree of self-actualization in simply being 'athletic' that leads to pride and self-respect. In order to reach this level, I'll quickly cover some of the basic ideas that are commonly adopted by coaches and athletes in the sports world. This will be enough to wrap one's head around the general practices that build athleticism.

Strength, power, and speed must be trained. Unlike other aspects of athleticism, these three central components will see more improvement by implementing a training routine than by simply playing sports. Strength and power are built most commonly by implementing a scalable program of compound lifting movements comprised mostly of barbell work. Perhaps the most popular and potent of these is Olympic weightlifting, which is one of the best platforms that we have for safe, scalable strength-building. It employs what we know about human biomechanics into a subset of lifting movements, primarily the snatch and the clean and jerk, but also the deadlift, squat, and other variations. It requires more mobility than other strength sports and builds power (explosive strength), which is a major component of overall athleticism. The modern day 'hack' of Olympic lifting, while only one hack among many, is a great example of how to leverage natural movement effectively, without resorting to mimicking actual natural movements (e.g. lifting logs or chasing a gazelle). But are there advantages to hunter-gatherer movements that are not captured fully by modern alternatives?

While it would be illogical to conclude that mimicking the natural movement patterns of hunter-gatherers would be an optimal fitness regimen, some argue that the physical adaptivity of truly natural movement is an effective route for developing athleticism, although difficult to recreate safely in the modern gym with contemporary equipment. For example, dragging a wide slippery log through the mud barefoot is actually a highly complex, adaptable maneuver involving not only the smooth cooperation of various physical processes (muscle coordination, balance, etc.) but also requiring the cognitive faculties of split-second judgment, adaptive foot and hand placement, tactile feedback, and self-protection. As you may imagine, this movement would require focus and the mental processing of multiple variables in order to complete the movement safely. Individuals may benefit from the challenge of complex movements like this, therefore developing overall athleticism more thoroughly. However, the more challenging the movement, the more dangerous it becomes.

Due to an increased likelihood of injury, highly complex training regimens may be unsuitable for athletes who need to minimize an already high risk of injury. At the other end of the spectrum, sensitive populations like the elderly do not require this level of intensity to see benefits. Normal folks should train many of these physical features (strength, stability, form, etc.), but they should do so in safe, scalable environment with the guidance of a professional.

Perhaps the most important anatomical feature of the athlete is the 'core', a group of muscles at the center of the athlete's body. The core includes the hips, buttocks, abdomen, lower back, and obliques. The core is the foundation of movement, because this is the power center of the body. It houses the largest muscle, the gluteus maximus (the butt), and all the muscles that keep the body upright, balanced, and stable.

The rest of the intangibles will come with training the athlete's particular skill, an idea captured by the coach's refrain: "Train the movement." If you want to get good at bowling, you have to throw bowling balls. Tennis, swing a racquet. There's no magic to the hard work and discipline necessary to build skill. It is as simple as dedicating oneself to deliberate practice.

Training the movement means guiding the body to adapt, and is a crucial concept in fitness because of its utility. The SAID principle, which stands for Specific Adaptations to Imposed Demands, states that the body will respond to stressors by adapting to meet the demands of those stressors. Moving weight, for instance, will stress the muscles, tendons, and joints; in turn, these will become stronger and tougher as a principle of adaptation. These adaptations clearly improve normal life, but only if they are functional. Bicep curls won't help much in, say, picking up a box, but deadlifts can. Bicep curls won't help as much in climbing as pull-ups. The body moves as one and training it that way can help. These are called complex movements, and include squats, deadlifts, overhead squats, the snatch, and many others where the whole body is engaged.

The Lost Art of Play

"Humanity has advanced, when it has advanced, not because it has been sober, responsible, and cautious, but because it has been playful, rebellious, and immature."
Tom Robbins, American author

As children, we play naturally without a second thought to its purpose. But this affectation to play is mostly lost in adults. While conventional wisdom may see that as an appropriate loss of childishness, it's important to ask: is there something to gain by reclaiming the spirit of play?

Everything we covered in the previous section was about working out to achieve fitness and athleticism. However, play is the antithesis of a workout. The opposite of work is rest, but the inverse of work is play. A workout is externally motivated and planned; play is intrinsically motivated and spontaneous. Workouts are intentionally tiring and mentally draining, even abusive; play ignites our energy and stirs our spirit. Workouts require willpower, discipline, and resolution; play is naturally free from those burdens. Just how natural is play? Stuart Brown is perhaps the foremost authority on play in humans. He is a medical doctor, psychiatrist, clinical researcher, and founder of the National Institute of Play. In his book about play, he outlines its evolutionary origins:

> Over time, as a result of a lengthening childhood play period, these primates learned to control their tendencies to dominate and fight, and began to be able to reconcile and care for each other. This is how they gained wisdom and survival skills. Those who missed out on play couldn't tell friend from foe, misread gestures, got rejected by potential mates, and floundered. The nonplayer didn't survive. Those who played survived, adapted, and developed skills and capabilities that their ancestors could never imagine.[180]

It's perhaps one of the most potent yet underappreciated topics in health. It's something that is undeniably natural, yet inscrutably lost. At certain ages and in countless scenarios, play is even stigmatized, looked down upon by the eyes of convention, pejoratively labeled as juvenile, despite its natural compulsions and the tremendous good it does the individual.

We may not be expected to play as adults, but we can still rebel against convention. We can invite others to join our antics, our lightened spirits resistant to the ugliness of the world, resilient against its monotony. We can be temporarily immune to the deadpan, the humorless. Play seems to be at the very heart of life and what it means to be alive. After all, to what avail is the businesslike way we conduct our relationships and run our lives? Perhaps Nietzsche said it best, "A man's maturity consists in having found again the

---

[180] Brown, Stuart. *Play: How it Shapes the Brain, Opens the Imagination, and Invigorates the Soul.* Penguin, 2010. p 197.

seriousness one had as a child, at play."

Children will lose themselves in play. They will become so engaged in their activities that time is suspended and their consciousness focused almost entirely on sensory experience. Connected to the world, they define for us the concept of 'flow'. As we will cover later, flow is a predictor — better, a mechanism — of happiness in the truest sense of the word. It is a form of well-being that is ancient and innate. And it's lost to many. Another victim of civilization.

Rediscovering play is as simple as finding a movement you enjoy. For most, this will be a movement that can be sustained until exhaustion. Personally, I can play disc golf for hours. I can hit a volleyball around with friends at the beach until I fall over laughing. I can dance the night away no matter what the DJ spins. Think about what makes you move and let it take you. Charles Bukowski once said, "Find what you love and let it kill you." There are countless passionate people who have done just that — and they all did it moving.

Barefooting

"Nike should make scissors you can run with."

Tim Siedell, comedian and Twitter phenom

If you go back far enough on the human timeline, our hominid pre-human ancestors were going about their lives totally barefoot. Their feet were more like hands and were vital to survival in the trees (ever wonder why humans have toes?). But somewhere along the line humans came down from the trees to live on the ground. The adaptive pressure for long toes faded as the adaptive pressure for bipedal balance, running, swimming, and maneuvering increased, ultimately leading to the shortening of the toes.[181]

---

[181] Rolian et al (2009). Walking, running, and the evolution of short toes in humans. *The Journal of Experimental Biology* 212: 713-721.

Eventually, humans did invent and employ minimalist shoes to aid travel and to ensure warmth, but for the most part relied on their bare feet to move.

Our early ancestors likely invented primitive footwear along with other tools necessary for survival. Though still going barefoot much of the time, sandals would have aided them in persistence hunts and rugged, unfamiliar terrain. Then, when our ancestors left Africa 60,000 years ago, they needed warm shoes to survive cold winters at higher latitudes. For these reasons, shoes were a part of human evolution for far longer than many recognize, although ancient forms of shoes were minimalist. They did not have air bubbles in the heel, for instance.

The importance of barefooting and primitive footwear to our ancestors leads to an important interpretation of shoes and lower leg development today. The soft-heeled shoes that are common actually leave our modern feet undeveloped, weak, and prone to injury. Soft shoes may provide comfort, but they interfere with natural, healthy stresses that lead to the strengthening of the arch and toes, the proper development of ligaments and tendons, and the learning of efficient foot placement, heel-toe interaction, and balance.

The critical time period during the development and strengthening of the lower leg is childhood. Increasingly, parents encourage their children to wear shoes that stagnate the foot's development and may even disfigure the feet and toes. Weak feet are prone to injury and discomfort. Orthotics are a temporary fix but only serve to further weaken the lower leg in the long run.

The case for barefooting is strongly supported scientifically. Harvard professor and researcher Daniel Lieberman has demonstrated that impact gradients (the measure of the force of impact) on the leg are significantly better for barefoot runners, who distribute the impact of their fall over time by landing on the forefoot and naturally allowing the leg to absorb the impact like a spring, unlike shod runners who strike first on the heel of their shoe, sending pronounced impact stresses up the entire leg and body.[182] The modern form of running, with the heel strike, is out of line with our evolved

---

[182] Lieberman et al (2010). Foot strike patterns and collision forces in habitually barefoot versus shod runners. *Nature* 463: 531-535.

biomechanics and may be the underlying cause of foot, leg, core, and back pain and injury.

Humans have been called 'the running ape' for good reason. It is one of the defining characteristics of our species' evolution. We are neither fast nor strong compared to other animals, but we have the distinct ability to run for extended periods of time thanks to the evolved systems of thermoregulation and bipedalism.[183] Thermoregulation is the ability of regulate heat. Our bodies are able to cool themselves due to sweat glands, which improve the cooling process by keeping our skin wet.[184] Most animals do not sweat, and must cool their bodies through breathing (panting). Some animals can't even control their breath. Their breathing is controlled subconsciously, like the human heartbeat. It's clear that the human body evolved in a way that was distinctive from other species, leading ultimately to a unique ability to run long distances.

We also evolved an advanced system of bipedalism. Not only can we balance on two feet easily, but our bodies make running highly efficient. Compared to our ancestor Australopithecus, we have short toes, a spring-like foot arch, a nuchal ligament, a long Achilles tendon, a narrow waist, and wide shoulders — all of which support more efficient biomechanics of running.[185] The evolved complexity inherent in our ability to run at the endurance level exhibits a survival advantage to do so at some point in the evolution of our species. Most likely, it was due to the necessity to find and obtain food.

Persistence hunting is a primitive style of hunting where the animal is given a lengthy chase until it finally dies of exhaustion. Unlike humans, prey animals do not possess the ability to sweat, and must regulate their heat through breathing. The breathing system is not as effective as the sweating system. Thus, we are able to literally chase an animal to death. Some tribes still practice persistence hunting today.

---

[183] Bramble and Lieberman (2004). Endurance running and the evolution of Homo. *Nature* 432: 345-352.

[184] Cheuvront and Haymes (2001). Thermoregulation and marathon running: a biological and environmental approach. *Sports Medicine* 31 (10): 743-762.

[185] Grine et al. *The First Humans: Origin and Early Evolution of the Genus Homo.* Springer, 2010: pp. 80.

Persistence hunting is like interval training and marathoning put together. The goal of the hunters is to keep the herd in sight by walking briskly and lightly jogging, occasionally speeding up to contain stray animals and herd them in the right direction. The popular running book, *Born to Run* by Christopher McDougall, concludes that long distance competition is natural, citing persistence running as evidence, but this isn't quite on the mark. Unlike the competitive Tarahumara of Mexico who race long distances at an impressive pace, our ancestors instead cooperated in the hunt, a marathon of intervals at various speeds, which is a better definition of what is natural based on persistence running. But how much is too much?

Perhaps a better question is, how much is enough? Most people don't need to see athletic levels of training in order to see improvements in health. Most people may even see damage at those levels, as many athletes do. Moderate levels of activity will provide benefits and avoid the costs of overtraining, especially if proper form is executed.

The forefoot strike is observed in traditional cultures where people run in thin sandals and leather shoes. It is also seen in children who naturally forefoot strike as they play. The biomechanics of our body are optimized for running a certain way, because of the evolutionary pressure to do so. A hunter with weak arches would have been unable to hunt, and may have found himself removed from the gene pool.

Many are surprised to learn that modern running was invented rather recently, largely due to the influence of the shoe company Nike during the 1970's jogging boom. This is when the athletic shoe market saw a dramatic increase in thick-heeled running shoes that were meant to be more comfortable than the relatively thin traditional shoes before them. To this day, competitive runners still train to some degree in their naked feet and compete in very thin shoes in order to improve balance, tactile feedback, and lower leg strength.

For the day-to-day runner or jogger, full barefooting may be unreasonable due to unknown terrain or unseen objects that can compromise safety. In order to provide the runner with some degree of protection from the elements while still encouraging a healthy forefoot strike, many companies have developed barefoot technologies consisting of all kinds of minimalist footwear, from sandals to closed-toe shoes. The most popular tend to be closed-toe shoes that blend in with the style of normal shoes, just without the thick heel. As it turns out, the thick heel is what encouraged the heel striking to begin with. Also, a shoe that fully encases the toes may be more suitable for athletic environments where toe injury is a risk (e.g. catching a toe on a rock).

Most recreational runners and joggers have been running the wrong way for much of their lives. They've been wearing soft-heeled shoes that hindered the full development of muscles, ligaments, bones, and joints of the lower leg. As such, it's important for a new runner transitioning into barefoot running to take it slow and scale their ambition over a matter of weeks in order to prevent injury. From my personal experience, it took over a year for my feet to fully strengthen, and they are still. As you progress in barefooting, you can expect to have improved balance and strength in your feet, and you will slowly increase your ability to navigate rough terrain.

Ultimately, going totally barefoot for long periods of time will help you to rediscover an important part of your body that has been cut off from the world. You will be able to engage with the textures of your surroundings on the sensitive pads of your feet, interacting with them in a new and ancient way. If you're anything like me, shoes will eventually become suffocating, like wearing gloves on a warm day, and you'll begin to crave the sensation of the world on the skin of your feet, as human ancestors have for millions of years.

Strategies in Natural Movement

Move for a better brain. Movement is critical to brain function, development, and health. It literally makes you smarter. How dumb are jocks again?

Emphasize moving naturally. The natural movements include walking, running, squatting, swimming, climbing, fighting, dancing, crawling, jumping, balancing, throwing, and lifting. Yoga, hiking, Pilates, parkour, gardening, martial arts, and many sports are great options.

Incorporate movement into your life. Start riding a bicycle to work or walking to the grocery store like so many of our grandparents did. It's movement apathy that kills us, the ceaseless sitting that destroys our health, degenerating the body and mind.

Go barefoot enough to build baseline strength. It doesn't have to be all day. A moderate amount of time spent barefoot will strengthen muscles, ligaments, skin, and tendons, and will help prevent fungal infections in skin and nails. Choose safe environments and wear shoes in dangerous environments where injury is a risk.

Train smart with scalable compound movements emphasizing strength, power, and speed. If it's your goal to get fit and your body can handle it, try barbell training, sprinting, metabolic conditioning, isometrics, or a related program. Always use professional guidance until you learn the ropes!

Train the movement. If you want to build a particular skill, dedicate yourself to deliberate practice. This is your brain mastering a movement.

Reclaim a spirit of play. If moving is fun, it'll be more sustainable, and better for your overall health. There are countless spontaneous moments passing us by. Seize them.

What's Up With Arm Dominance?

There are clues all around us as to how we evolved based on the necessity of the evolved trait. Have you ever noticed that the vast majority of people today tend to favor one arm over the other for activities such as writing or throwing a ball? The necessity to specialize with one arm is true today just as it was for our ancestors. Ancient remains reveal teeth marks that suggest many of our ancient ancestors were right-handed.[186] The bones of the right arm are more heavily muscled with thicker ligaments and tendons, a strong indicator of the use of that arm. Right-handedness may have developed parallel to our ancestors' need to communicate, since both of these things are housed in the left-dominant brain.[187]

Achieving Natural Posture

Good posture has always been promoted, but never clearly defined. They tell us to 'stand tall' or 'stand up straight', but what exactly does that mean? With an evolutionary perspective, we can go beyond just 'standing up straight' to determining the proper mechanics of the hips, spine, and shoulders, proper breathing habits and bending movements — as they were designed by nature. Be assured that this is one topic the mainstream has gotten way wrong.

It's conventionally held that a normal spine forms an 'S' that snakes up our torso. The lumbar region is supposed to curve inward while the thoracic region curves outward. The problem with the word

---

[186] Frayer et al (2012). 500,000 years of right-handedness in Europe. *Laterality* 17(1).

[187] Corballis, Michael C (2003). From mouth to hand: gesture, speech, and the evolution of right-handedness. *Behavioral and Brain Sciences* 26: 199-208.

'normal' is that it's based on norms. And norms are rarely optimal. In fact, the 'normal' back has pain, tightness, and some likelihood of injury. Clearly, this is not a goal to be strived for.

The S-curve has its roots in modernity. Our day-to-day lives do not require natural movement that retains the proper alignment of our spines. Instead, we perform chronic tasks while sitting, and exercise on treadmills and bikes that only aid the deterioration of posture. Think about the countless young adults that ruin their posture with heavy backpacks.

Yet the 'normal' S-curve has permeated our culture, only adding to the problem. Our chairs are designed for this type of back curve. Our doctors see nothing wrong with it. Our beds and pillows are meant to cater to an S-curve that has no evolutionary precedence, an S-curve that results in back and neck problems down the road and skirts the benefits of a truly natural spine.

An evolutionary perspective on posture is limited, because this is a field that has gone largely unexplored. However, it seems obvious that an examination of traditional societies around the world would be insightful, because these are populations that maintain healthy backs their entire lives without pain or injury. A leading figure in the field of back health is Esther Gokhale, a back pain specialist with an anthropological perspective. Formally trained in acupuncture and biochemistry, Gokhale spent years studying the posture and movement of primal cultures that were devoid of back pain, ultimately developing her own method of treating it.

Some of the key concepts behind achieving a more natural posture are:

- **It's a J-curve, not an S-curve.** A true spine forms more of a J, where the bottom part of the J is your butt sticking out, and your upper spine is flat up all the way through the neck. Years of sitting unnaturally, carrying backpacks, staring at computers, etc., are the likely culprit of our poor modern posture.

- **Stand up straight and stick out your butt a little.** A bent-over posture looks timid. Not only does standing naturally make you a tiny bit taller, but it also allows you to exude confidence, health, and, in turn, attractiveness. It's also better for all your working parts, allowing safe movement and proper muscle development while avoiding injury.

- **Use your inner corset.** Experiment with lightly wrapping your core muscles to form a tight cylinder around your stomach and lower back. If breathing is impeded, you're wrapping too tightly. Instead, tighten your obliques while relaxing the rectus abdominus (the front of the stomach).

- **Breathing is an essential part of your posture.** In fact, breathing will change the size and structure of your rib cage. People are told all kinds of things regarding proper breathing patterns, but anthropological observations are clear: natural breathing is a combination of stomach, chest, and upper back. Go ahead and play around to find your comfort zone.

- **Hinge at the hip.** Bending should not change the 'core' of your back. Simply hinge at the hip rather than the waist.

Here's an exercise that may help you achieve optimal posture: While standing, raise your hands in front to elbow height while leaving the elbows in place, then move your hands slowly away from each other while breathing in slowly, filling your stomach mostly, and your chest and back, all the while imagining that the top of your head is being pulled skyward. Feel yourself get taller and taller, and then let the air fall out of your chest while maintaining the position in your back and stomach. Repeat. Then drop your hands, breathe freely, and feel the straight line of your spine and the firmness in your core.

What's the Natural Way to...um...Poop?

Believe it or not, sitting atop the porcelain throne is not how humans evolved to defecate. Humans naturally poop by squatting all the way down on their haunches. Unfortunately, partly due to the convenience and comfort of the toilet, some people lose their ability to perform this basic movement. On the other hand, many people who seek relief from poop-related disease take up the traditional squat in order to use their parts more naturally. It isn't for everyone, but it does make sense.

"If sleep does not serve an absolutely vital process, then it is the biggest mistake the evolutionary process has ever made."

Allan Rechtschaffen

pioneer of sleep research, psychologist, University of Chicago

CHAPTER 5

MAXIMIZING SLEEP QUALITY FOR MOOD, PRODUCTIVITY, AND HEALING

In 1893, the people of the world were swept up in a gleaming spectacle of history. The great city of Chicago transformed itself into a bustling metropolis as people flocked from afar, ready to exhibit for the world the front lines of progress and technological revolution. All around them at the world's fair, the future shined on their skin and filled their eyes on a scale that had never been known before.

The Columbian Exposition, a world's fair celebrating the 400th anniversary of the discovery of the New World, occurred at the peak of the rivalry between Thomas Edison and Nikola Tesla, who were each vying to popularize their electrical inventions, direct current and alternating current, respectively. In the end, Tesla won the bid to light the exposition and the world saw for the first time the potential of this new technology, but not its implications. What they witnessed was the end of night as humans have known it for millions of years.

The exposition was held on 600 acres and featured 200 buildings, showing the world that Chicago had risen from the devastating fires of 1871. It reached an attendance in record numbers, drawing 716,881 people. It was ripe with products and ideas that still exist today, names like Pabst Blue Ribbon, Cream of Wheat, and Juicy Fruit. The first Ferris Wheel turned high in the air. It was a momentous occasion for America and for the world, exhibiting a commitment to innovation and prosperity, a dedication to progress, and a love for technology. It was an occasion to be proud of, even today. Understanding its historical weight helps us to see the social and cultural environment that led to new technologies. The sobering reality, though, is that the people witnessing this spectacle of history were blind to the impact it would have on public health and society.

What is Sleep Anyway?

Sleep remains one of the great unsolved mysteries of nature. Precisely why we sleep and the role sleep plays is of particular importance to researchers and remains a vital area of study today. Likewise, the evolutionary perspective yields a dissonant interpretation that represents many conflicting views about how exactly our prehistoric ancestors behaved during the night.

Sleep at first doesn't seem to make sense in terms of evolution. Since animals are unconscious while they sleep, they would seem to be vulnerable to predators (or friends with permanent markers!). Predators before 10,000 years ago were nothing to shake a stick at — we're talking about saber-tooth tigers, ferocious packs of dire wolves, giant bears, and 27-foot crocodiles. But it isn't as simple as predators and prey, because humans have long been apex predators themselves, and sleep is a biological necessity.

Evolution tells a different story about night vulnerability. Early human ancestors likely slept in the protection of trees until finally descending to the savannah upon the discovery of fire. Richard Wrangham, anthropologist at Harvard, writes,

> Homo erectus presumably climbed no better than modern humans do, unlike the agile habilines [homo habilis]. This shift suggests that Homo erectus slept on the ground, a novel

behavior that would have depended on their controlling fire to provide light to see predators and scare them away.[188]

The presence of predators on the ground were no doubt a danger, but even among fearsome predators of the Paleolithic, our species was also an apex predator of the savanna, and was simply not the natural prey of many of these large predators, who would understandably prefer to hunt big, dumb, delicious bison over packs of bony, clever, weapon-bearing humans. Even today, humans are feared by other predators due to the power of our tools, our control of fire, and our strength in numbers. This fact mitigates the dangers of sleeping at night and offers clues as to our natural sleep rhythms.

Sleep may also be a biological necessity as a recurring state of repair and healing. All mammals and birds sleep in some way, shape, or form. Sleep deprivation studies on humans affect behavior and physiology.[189] Studies also show that sleep deprivation negatively affects cognition.[190] Mood can also be subject to sleep loss, increasing irritability, pessimism, and depression.[191] All of the negative effects of sleep loss would affect one's physical ability, interaction with others, decision making, etc., all things that affect survivability in the wild. Thus, sleep would have retained its evolutionary role in nature simply as a matter of survival.

Anthropological observations on modern hunter-gatherer tribes and those removed from technology reveal different kinds of sleeping patterns. People tend to sleep when they like, according to their culture. Some sleep in two or more phases per day or night, while others sleep in one solid session. But for modern humans, many of us are restricted to an 8-hour window that

---

[188] Wrangham, R. *Catching Fire: How Cooking Made Us Human.* New York: Basic Books, 2009.

[189] Banks S, Dinges DF (2007). Behavioral and physiological consequences of sleep restriction. *Journal of Clinical Sleep Medicine* 3: 519–528.

[190] Van Dongen HP, Maislin G, Mullington JM, Dinges DF (2003). The cumulative cost of additional wakefulness: Dose-response effects on neurobehavioral functions and sleep physiology from chronic sleep restriction and total sleep deprivation. *Sleep* 26: 117–126.

[191] Peterson and Benca (2006). Sleep in mood disorders. *Psychiatric Clinics of North America* 29(4):1009-1032.

is squeezed tightly within the demands of our lives. The strategy, then, becomes to optimize that sleeping window best we can.

One major influence on sleep patterns is light, particularly the way it affects our hormones. Our skin and eyes have evolved to interact intricately with the light energy around us.[192] Throughout time in the wild, we slept according to the sun — that is, the fluctuation of light and dark. So it only makes sense that sunlight would play an important role in our bodies. We know that it does for nutrition (vitamin D from UVB rays), but the same is true for hormonal regulation according to the light that interacts with our eyes and falls on our skin.

One vital connection is cortisol, a potent hormone generated by the adrenal gland. It is released as a response to stress and activates gluconeogenesis (the formation of blood sugar). Therefore, it plays a role in regulating energy levels, carrying further implications explored in Chapter 3 on human diet. Our bodies naturally regulate cortisol production according to day-night patterns. At night, cortisol levels are low in order to allow our bodies to sleep. In the day, they are elevated in order to stabilize energy levels and moderate immune function. But cortisol is elevated when sleep times are low,[193] which further disturbs the quality of sleep and even the ability to sleep. Cortisol works in concert with increasing levels of melatonin and adenosine, which help to bring about sleep. Since these hormones and molecules also depend on light levels, they too are at risk of imbalance in an environment that signals lengthened days.

Hormonal rhythms are affected by recent modern technology. The trouble began with the popularization of artificial lighting since the 1800s. It was a momentous achievement of the Industrial Revolution, but it effectively brought about the end of 'night'. Today, lighting technology is nearly universal and has significantly extended the 'daytime' as our bodies perceive it. These 'long days' throw off the complex biochemical cascades (cortisol,

---

[192] Borbely AA (1982) A two process model of sleep regulation. *Human Neurobiology* 1: 195–204.

[193] Leproult et al (1997). Sleep loss results in the elevation of cortisol levels the next evening. *Sleep* 20(10): 865-870.

melatonin, adenosine) that govern sleep patterns and, with a medley of other problems like poor diet and stress, ultimately impact sleep quantity and sleep quality to a significant degree. In turn, this feedback loop can exacerbate disease and significantly decrease quality of life.

Studies show that getting less than 8 hours of sleep a day can compromise the immune system,[194] cause drowsiness and stress, augment appetite,[195] impair memory,[196] exacerbate aging,[197] and lead to metabolic syndrome[198] (obesity and diabetes). Yet, the role sleep plays in augmenting health and curtailing disease is currently underappreciated in modern culture. Sayings like "Sleep is for the weak" pervade many competitive settings, only serving to further downplay an essential biological function — one that requires about a third of our lifetimes!

While remembering the fallacy that mimicking the natural sleep patterns of our ancestors is optimal, there is enormous potential to hack our sleep. Evolved hormonal mechanisms govern all kinds of functions in the body, and they are all related to sleep quality and sleep quantity. The health benefits to sleeping better include improving body weight, lowering stress, controlling appetite, normalizing blood pressure, elevating mood, reversing type-2 diabetes, protecting against heart disease, restoring energy, and minimizing cancer risk.[199]

The most important way to take advantage of our evolved light-detection mechanisms is to control the light around us according to sleep times. This can be done with the use of blackout curtains. These will restrict light to the

[194] Penelope et al (2004). Sick and tired: does sleep have a vital role in the immune system? *Nature Reviews Immunology* 4: 457-467.

[195] Spiegel et al (2004). Sleep curtailment in healhty young men is associated with decreased leptin levels, increased ghrelin levels, and increase hunger and appetite. 141 (11): 846-850.

[196] Diekelmann and Born (2010). The memory function of sleep. *Nature Reviews Neuroscience* 11:114-126.

[197] Spiegel et al (1999). Impact of sleep debt on metabolic and endocrine function. The Lancet 354(9188): 1435-1439.

[198] Cauter et al (2008). Metabolic consequences of sleep and sleep loss. Sleep Medicine 9 (1): S23-S28.

[199] Wiley, TS. *Lights Out: Sleep, Sugar, and Survival.* New York: Pocket Books, 2000.

bedroom, allowing a more perfect darkness suitable for sleeping, no matter the time of day or night. Even the smallest traces of faint light hitting our skin can affect hormonal regulation, so it's a good idea to augment blackout curtains by taping off the small power lights of laptops, outlets, and other electronic devices. Perfect darkness is the goal because it allows undisturbed sleep rhythms until waking. In effect, blackout curtains are a way of shortening the artificially 'long day' by lengthening the artificial night.

Here is a long list of commonly and not-so-commonly used sleep strategies that may or may not work for you:

- Aim for 8-10 hours of sleep a night.
- Eat a whole foods diet to keep toxins out of the body that hinder sleep quality.
- Make sure you're tired when you go to bed by exercising daily.
- Get blackout curtains to keep the room as dark as possible.[200]
- Supplement with magnesium an hour before bed to set the biological clock.[201]
- Supplement with omega-3 in order to promote healing.[202]
- Restrict caffeine to the early morning, or quit altogether.[203] [204]
- Keep the room temperature cool (~65 degrees).
- Avoid overeating close to bedtime.
- Sleep when tired, wake naturally without an alarm.

---

[200] Durlach et al (2002). Biorhythms and possible central regulation fo magnesium status, phototherapy, darkness therapy, and chronopathological forms of magnesium depletion. *Magnesium Research* 15(1-2):49-66.

[201] Durlach et al (2002). Chronopathological forms of magnesium depletion with hypofunction or with hyperfunction of the biological clock. *Magnesium Research* 15(3-4):263-8.

[202] Stevens et al (1996). Omega-3 fatty acids in boys with behavior, learning, and health problems. *Physiology and Behavior* 59 (4-5): 915–920.

[203] Brezinova, Blasta (1974). Effect of caffeine on sleep. *British Journal of Clinical Pharmacology* 1 (3): 203-208.

[204] Landolt et al (1995). Caffeine reduces low-frequency delta activity in human sleep EEG. *Neuropsychopharmacology* 12 (3): 229-238.

- Avoid late night liquids that would cause a middle-of-the-night bathroom trip.
- Turn off cell phones and beeping watches.
- Use a sleep mask when traveling.
- Wind down with something imaginative like a work of fiction.
- Wake at the same time each day.

Is Snoring an Evolved Trait?

When interpreting evolution, we have to keep in mind that certain traits that have manifested in our species, in this case snoring, may or may not be advantageous in survival terms. This is the trouble in finding a definitive conclusion, because some things in biology are admittedly perplexing. However, this fact does not hinder the fun of interpretation. On one hand, snoring could have easily attracted unwanted attention. However, humans were not the natural prey of many of the predators of the savannah, and it's likely that tribes employed some loose form of night watch or at the very least kept a fire blazing that would have scared off any threats.

So how could snoring be an evolutionary advantage? If you listen to snoring, it's a rather aggressive sound, like the snarl of a dog. For a wandering creature, the sound may be enough to scare them off, and it certainly would be enough to denote to the creature that whoever made the sound was awake. Whatever the case, like much of evolutionary interpretation, this answer is not definitive.

Ocular Adaptation

The human eye has the ability to adjust to various levels of

---

darkness and light. It is referred to in ocular physiology as adaptation, and is enabled by the rods and cones of the eye. Obviously, vision is important to survival, yet compared to many other animals, our night vision is not very effective. It takes 20-30 minutes for our eyes to fully adjust to darkness, and even then our night vision isn't impressive. There are animals that can see both farther and more clearly at night than we can in the day. Human vision is optimized to daylight hours, necessitated by daily activities such as hunting, etc. This means that we are a diurnal (daytime) species. And that 20-30 minutes it takes to adapt to changing light levels is an interesting figure, because that's about how long it takes for the sun to rise and set. It's almost like we evolved that way or something.

"Everything is amazing and nobody is happy."

Louis CK

everyman comedian

CHAPTER 6

REVEALING EVOLVED

PATHWAYS TO HAPPINESS

You may not know it, but you have won the evolutionary lottery. Statistically speaking, you have won the lottery many times over. If you consider the myriad directions, the endless possibilities that life could have taken as it slowly evolved over time, facing extinctions and coming to terms with the brutality of nature, it is truly miraculous that we arrived where we are now as humans. We could have been the slithering serpent, a deadly bacterium, or any ignoble organism, a droplet in the oceans of life. Instead, we are intelligent, moral, and happy. Or are we?

According to the Centers for Disease Control and Prevention, 1 in 10 US adults report depression. Over a hundred Americans will commit suicide today, the great majority of them males.[205] These are extreme examples, but what about the other end of the spectrum, where the lost and wandering souls of the world do not fit neatly into such statistical boundaries? There are the

---

[205] American Association of Suicidology. *U.S.A. Suicide: 2010 Official Data.* [PDF file] Retrieved from http://www.suicidology.org/c/document_library/get_file?folderId=262&name=DLFE-636.pdf

lonely, the chronically stressed, the pathological, the ill, the miserable. Henry David Thoreau famously said, "The mass of men lead lives of quiet desperation," and not-so-famously said in the same passage, "...it is a characteristic of wisdom not to do desperate things." How do we account for the desperate? The lost? The empty? The anguished? Can this be solved? How are we even happy to begin with?

The picture of humanity in the wild is certainly not one of utopia. Life was rugged. Yet according to the evolutionary pressures of the environment, our species nevertheless evolved a complex set of emotions.[206] Many of these emotions are positive — joy, love, play, euphoria, ecstasy, pleasure, gratification, satisfaction, triumph, amusement, you name it — all of which are an intrinsic part of the human animal, and are loosely captured scientifically and otherwise by one loaded word: happiness. Generally defined, happiness is a mental or emotional state of well-being characterized by positive emotions ranging from contentment to intense joy and beyond. Researchers use all kinds of words with nuanced definitions and differences, words like "life satisfaction," "fulfillment," and "well-being."

One of the revelatory facts of evolution is that nature selected for these traits in humans. It's marvelous to consider how humans, like many other animals, are naturally playful, pleasure-seeking, and positive. These are the things that arose out of a callous world based on survival. Thanks to evolution, we are happy. And thanks to science, we now know enough about happiness than ever before, giving us the opportunity to lead more fulfilling lives.

Back to Basics

One simple framework for thinking about the components of happiness is an old model commonly resurfacing in psychology called the Hierarchy of

---

[206] Darwin, Charles (1872). *The expression of the emotions in man and animals.* New York: Filiquarian, 2007.

Needs. You've probably heard of it. It was first proposed by Abraham Maslow in 1943 and then later published fully in 1954 in the book *Motivation and Personality*. Maslow followed what he called "exemplary people" and identified the basic human needs for which these people strived. Then, he ranked them in order of importance:

1. **Physiological needs**: breathing, food, water, sex, sleep, excretion.

2. **Safety**: security of employment, resources, family, health, property.

3. **Belonging**: love, friendship, family, emotional and sexual intimacy.

4. **Esteem**: self-esteem, confidence, achievement, respect of others.

5. **Self-actualization**: morality, creativity, spontaneity, lack of prejudice, problem solving, acceptance of facts.[207]

This model is often presented as a pyramid with the physiological needs at the base and self-actualization at the top, although Maslow himself did not present it that way. The pyramid is a helpful metaphor of building upon one's needs in order to fulfill them. By extension, these things directly contribute to human happiness, making Maslow's hierarchy a useful tool for analyzing life fulfillment.

During most of its history, the field of psychology has been devoted to understanding mental illness: depression, anxiety, neurosis, etc. Like medicine today, it was permeated by a pessimistic view of human nature, that man was inherently flawed and needed fixing. In 1998, Martin Seligman became president of the American Psychology Association and shared a radical new vision for the future of the field of psychology. He urged fellow researchers to "turn toward understanding and building the human strengths to complement our emphasis on healing damage." Rather than working toward making sick people normal, Seligman noted the value of working toward making normal people better. He recognized this as a part of the field that had gone

---

[207] Maslow, Abraham. (1954) *Motivation and Personality*. HarperCollins, 1987.

unexplored. In the words of Martin Seligman, 'positive psychology' seeks to attain a scientific understanding of "positive human functioning" with the goal of "making normal life more fulfilling". This idea echoes the discord hypothesis, because normal life, as we understand it to mean in civilization, is so clearly out of line with human nature. Can questioning the merit of "normal life" lead us to see human well-being more clearly?

In contemporary society, normal people are not happy. Normal people have sabotaged almost every layer of their fundamental needs, starting with the most important: health. The normal person today is not healthy in strict terms. They may be temporarily disease-free, but more often than not they are unfit, sleep-deprived, stressed, and malnourished. Normal people experience job stress yet also worry about money. Many come from broken nuclear families, or have lost touch with their closest friends. Normal people struggle with body image and self-esteem. These things hinder happiness because they do not overcome the challenges of society. The attitude that normal is good distracts us from the truth that we can do better. This isn't to say that civilization is bad, only that some of it is.

The vast range of human emotion is a real and valuable part of human life. Psychologist Kay Redfield Jamison proclaimed, "If I can't feel, if I can't move, if I can't think, and I can't care, then what conceivable point is there in living?"[208] She wrote these words in the context of manic-depression, a condition that highlights the vast range of human emotion. Within the context of society, our range is fully taxed in day-to-day life. While things like depression may not seem to make sense within an evolutionary framework (good luck reproducing after suicide), the vast range of human emotion is real. Our nature is one of conscious exuberance, embedded in thinking, feeling, and interacting. It is a defining characteristic of the human experience, a gift of nature.

In 2002 and 2012, geneticist and evolutionary biologist Bjørn Grinde published and then updated *Darwinian Happiness: Evolution as a Guide for Living*

---

[208] Jamison, Kay R. *An Unquiet Mind: a memoir of moods and sadness.* New York: Vintage Books, 1995.

and Understanding Human Behavior. In this book, he lays groundwork for an evolutionary and biological interpretation of positive and negative emotions. In evolutionary terms, emotions arise due to the survival advantage that they offer the individual. Evolution explains how humans seek out positive things (friendship, community, food, etc.) and avoid negative things (pain, injury, danger), and demonstrates how this affects survivability. Grinde argues that we should, as modern humans, strive toward emphasizing those positive associations and avoiding the negative ones.

Grinde notes that many of the living conditions that arise from modernity directly vie with human nature in ways that cause unhappiness. In his review of the book, published in the *Journal of Evolutionary Psychology*, Peter Crabb notes:[209]

- The absence of parents in the day-to-day lives of children may adversely affect their psychopathological development.

- The culture of obsessive cleanliness and sterility may adversely affect the development of the immune system, weakening the body against disease.

- Oppressive sexual mores can stifle emotional intimacy, bonding, and sexual expression. On the other hand, an unprecedented availability of potential sexual partners can lead to fractured relationships and broken families.

- City-living in general is a discord with our past, and causes a host of problems.[210]

The interpretation of how we lived then and now can spiral into vast layers of detail and conjecture, and conclusions about what to do depend greatly on the goals of the individual. So where can we start in order to shed light on human happiness? What characterizes the happiness of our species and underlies mental well-being? The answer lies in our most potent evolved trait, one that granted us strength in the wild and ultimately led to the tapestry

---

[209] Crabb, Peter (2003). Stalking the Good Life. *Journal of Evolutionary Psychology* 1:158-160.

[210] Morris, Desmond. *The Human Zoo: a zoologist's study of the urban animal.* New York: Kodansha Globe, 1996.

of society in which we live today.

The Social Animal

"The Way of Men is the way of the gang."

Jack Donovan, American author

Human beings are arguably the most social creatures that evolution has ever produced. Our social structures are the most complex in the animal kingdom. Our bonds are arguably the deepest. Our emotions are the most varied and nuanced. All thanks to the evolutionary environment. This sociality gave us strength against the dangers, the hardships, and the chaos. But in civilization, this sociality is compromised. The dangers are replaced with comforts, the hardships with inconveniences, and the chaos with routine, dampening the civilized person's sense of belonging, social standing, and connection with others.

For scientists in the world of happiness, positive social interaction is king. It's perhaps the most consistently positive instigator of happiness and may be the most glaring inconsistency between the way we evolved and the way we live today. As reported by *Time* magazine:

> A 2002 study conducted at the University of Illinois by Diener and Seligman found that the most salient characteristics shared by the 10% of students with the highest levels of happiness and the fewest signs of depression were their strong ties to friends and family and commitment to spending time with them. "Word needs to be spread," concludes Diener. "It is important to work on social skills, close interpersonal ties and social support in order to be happy."[211]

---

[211] Wallis, Claudia (2005). "The New Science of Happiness." *Time Magazine.* Retrieved from http://www.time.com/time/magazine/article/0,9171,1015902-1,00.html

Compared to how we evolved, humans today do not spend the quantity or quality of time in positive social engagement. As they say, life happens. Culture and the dictates of society have overcome the value we place on friends, family, social networks, and community. More and more, people are spending their leisure time in solitary activities.[212] Even recent generations are seeing this trend toward isolation.[213] With this shift in our cultural value system comes a lifestyle that does not fully utilize our evolved mechanisms of happiness. However, we can tap the potential for these mechanisms simply by recognizing them and employing a strategy.

If positive social interaction is the goal, then the strategy is to find love, aggregate friends, and build a sense of community. That means nurturing regular contact with family and committing yourself to a tight network of quality friends and mentors. And it means doing so with *intention*. The previously mentioned study by Diener and Seligman highlights the "commitment" these individuals had to investing time in their friends and family. In the wild, our ancestors had no choice but to spend significant time with loved ones. In civilization, we have a choice, so we must recognize the importance of identifying appropriate people to engage with and taking strides to share time and deepen bonds with them.

While we respond strongly to the positive, human beings are especially sensitive to negative inputs, whether those be a rude person or a bitter tasting food. Nancy Etcoff, an evolutionary psychologist and cognitive researcher, explains that humans evolved sensitivity to negatives as a matter of survival. She explains, "Our taste buds react more strongly to bitter tastes than to sweet ones. That might help us avoid poison."[214] Extending the idea to social interactions, Etcoff cites research on successful marriages that have observed

---

[212] Putnam, Joseph (1995). "Bowling alone: America's Declining Social Capital." *Journal of Democracy.* 134-142.

[213] McPherson, Smith-Lovin, and Brashears (2006). Social Isolation in America: Changes in Core Discussion Networks Over Two Decades. *American Sociological Review* 71 (3): 353-375.

[214] Lambert, Craig. "The Science of Happiness." *Harvard Magazine.* Feb., 2007. Retrieved from http://harvardmagazine.com/2007/01/the-science-of-happiness.html

couples using a ratio of 5 to 1 positive-negative gestures while arguing. Etcoff believes this demonstrates to some degree the scale of potency for positive and negative interaction — that is, negative interactions are five times more potent than positive ones. Therefore, avoiding negative social interaction can be just as important as, if not more important, than encouraging positive social interaction. As Chuck Palahniuk once said, "It's so hard to forget pain, but it's even harder to remember sweetness. We have no scar to show for happiness. We learn so little from peace."

Much of happiness are the things that govern our wants and our likes, things that depend on our biological signals. While not to discount the role that culture and social factors play in the formation and expression of feeling and emotion,[215] in order for happiness to be an evolved trait, it must be hardwired to our biological systems via heritable characteristics in order to be selected for by nature. This is in fact the case, as confirmed by neuroscience, due to our hard-wired reward/motivation pathways.[216] Dopamine is a neurotransmitter that plays a major role in our brain's reward/motivation system.[217] Serotonin is another neurotransmitter that regulates mood, appetite, sleep, and plays a role in memory and learning. Oxytocin is the "love hormone" that plays a role in arousal, orgasm, empathy, and bonding. The sex hormones, estrogen and testosterone, play a role in libido and arousal in both men and women. Together, these are the central characters in the reward and pleasure systems that are at the heart of our evolved likes, wants, and desires.

As social animals, it should be clear that positive engagement with others affects these biological pathways. Cooperation, for instance, affects the reward centers of the brain, and has been shown to induce reward in humans.[218] This

[215] Davidson, RJ. (2001). Toward a Biology of Personality and Emotion. *Annals of the New York Academy of Sciences* 935: 191–207.

[216] Genetic Science Learning Center (1969). Beyond the Reward Pathway. *Learn.Genetics.* Retrieved May 18, 2012, from
http://learn.genetics.utah.edu/content/addiction/reward/pathways.html

[217] Salamone and Correa (2012). The mysterious motivational functions of mesolimbic dopamine. *Neuron* 76 (3): 470.

[218] Krill and Platek (2012). Working together may be better: activation of reward centers during

is in line with the 'social brain hypothesis', which states that human brains are naturally hardwired for cooperation with others in a way that augments evolutionary success. Some believe that advancements in the human brain may have been due to the demands of forming intimate pair bonds, not simply due to the demands of living in complex social networks.[219] A study out of the University of Michigan in 2010 demonstrates the activation of the brain reward center when testing reciprocity among cooperating adults.[220] The perception of fairness in their dealings led to rewards on the neurological level, which may be the fundamental framework for establishing trust and maintaining social relationships, further growing the human brain. The link between cooperation and survival is certainly in line with evolutionary theory, and sends a strong message about the nature of our species given that cooperation itself is so closely tied to the architecture of the brain.

The Science of Happiness

In 2005, Nobel Prize-winning psychologist Daniel Kahneman of Princeton University unveiled a new method of measuring happiness called the day-reconstruction method. Participants filled out a long diary and questionnaire, noting who they were with and rating the experience on a seven point scale. It was tested on 900 women in Texas. Top activities for happiness included sex, socializing, praying/meditating, and eating. In light of evolution, does praying seem out of place?

Not according to George Valliant, who argues that the satisfaction inherent to religious faith is a part of human nature. In his own words, "Mammalian evolution has hard-wired the brain for spiritual experience."[221]

---

cooperative maze task. *PLoS One* 7 (2): e30613.

[219] Dunbar and Schultz (2007). Evolution in the social brain. *Science* 317 (5843): 1344-1347.

[220] Phan et al (2010). Reputation for reciprocity engages the brain reward center. *Proceedings of the National Academy of Sciences* 107 (29): 13099-13104.

[221] Lambert, Craig. The Science of Happiness. *Harvard Magazine* [Web file] Retrieved from http://harvardmagazine.com/2007/01/the-science-of-happiness.html

Many studies link religion and happiness closely. It's unclear whether the idea of God or the church community are the causal factors, but it's likely some combination of both.

Religion can also be a manifestation of our need for security. Just as Maslow's Needs underscore our need for security of employment, safety, and health, the need to feel safe for one's soul after death (as well as the souls of loved ones) can become an important factor in the human mind, helping to put it at ease and feel good about its future, no matter how distant or unlikely.[222] This, in turn, can affect happiness levels by both relieving anxiety over the uncertainty of death and creating positive anticipation for the future of the individual.

Evolutionary theory also explains why human beings are compassionate, despite popular presumptions that we are selfish. Ironically, our compassion may be due to our selfishness. Biologists point out that individuals often favor their kin consciously, and that this might have been due to the survival advantage to do so. When we are driven to help someone related to us, we are actually helping our own genes survive, based on the fact that the family shares the same genetic heritage. Since favoring our kin would help our genes carry on through time, 'kin selection' (or nepotistic altruism) may have been the survival advantage that spurred a layer of compassion toward family members, since positive emotions towards these people would provide an evolutionary advantage to shared genetic material. However, compassion existed long before the dawn of humans.

This may explain why we developed compassion for our family, but what about the other members of our tribe or strangers? Compassion developed further with the concept of 'reciprocal altruism', which explains how helping others in various ways creates reciprocity among members of a group as long as individuals manage the incentives of cooperation through threat and punishment. In this cooperative environment, the cooperating individuals would increase the group's odds of survival and therefore increase each

---

[222] Vail et al (2010). A terror management analysis of the psychological functions of religion. *Personality and Social Psychology Review* 14 (1): 84-94.

individual's odds of survival.[223] Reciprocal altruism sheds light on the advantage of compassion.

What remains, however, is compassion for strangers, which seems to lack an evolutionary explanation. Robert Wright explains that in the real world, we are far more compassionate toward those within our own social network than those outside of it.[224] Despite the fact that we may retain some marginal degree of compassion for strangers, there exists significantly more compassion for our social network and, to an even greater degree, our families. From an evolutionary perspective, this makes sense. Strangers were rare in the ancestral environment, and those that interacted with our ancestors did not augment reproductive fitness as significantly as our social networks or families.

'Group selection' has become the buzzword recently that has gained popularity as evolutionists seek to reveal how living in groups affected human evolution. The idea is part of multi-level evolution, which explains how selfless genetic traits have appeared in humans. Many people demonstrate an inherent will to offer individual sacrifices for others, expecting nothing in return. It is believed that group selection explains this phenomenon. However, Steven Pinker has refined this understanding, pointing out that 'group selection' is simply a metaphor for the gene-level selection of the individual within a group:

> If a person has innate traits that encourage him to contribute to the group's welfare and as a result contribute to *his own* welfare, group selection is unnecessary; individual selection in the context of group living is adequate.[225]

---

[223] Trivers, Robert L (1971). "The Evolution of Reciprocal Altruism." *The Quarterly Review of Biology* 46 (1): 35-57.

[224] Wright, Robert. (2008). "The Evolution of Compassion." [Video file]. Retrieved from http://www.ted.com/talks/lang/en/robert_wright_the_evolution_of_compassion.html.

[225] Pinker, Steven (2012). The false allure of group selection. *Edge Magazine*. Retrieved from http://edge.org/conversation/the-false-allure-of-group-selection.

Thus, 'group selection' is a helpful idea for thinking through the group dynamics of human evolution, but is nevertheless limited and mechanized by the classic understanding of human evolution, which takes places at the individual's genetic level.

Martin Seligman, the pioneer of positive psychology, prefers to outline three basic forms of the happy life that seek to move beyond the evolutionary model.[226] First is the 'pleasant life', which is characterized by simple and heightened pleasures such as eating good food, smiling, enjoying wine, going on vacation, or having sex. The pleasant life is perhaps the most concrete interpretation of human happiness. Indeed, for most people, this is the type of happiness most commonly pursued. But Seligman notes that pleasantries do not necessarily lead to life satisfaction.

The 'good life' is one outside the realm of pleasure, characterized by engagement with the world and our surroundings. An important component is 'flow', a common topic in the field of positive psychology.[227] It describes a positive mental state of full immersion and energized focus in an activity. The activity may be work or play, but it is the concept of flow that elevates these activities to characterize what Seligman calls the good life. In flow, time is suspended, and the individual achieves a great sense of connection with the world, the activities that engage them, and the people around them.

Finally, Seligman outlines the 'meaningful life' as the highest form of happiness. This is characterized by higher duty, strength of character, excellence, and virtue. In a newsletter, Seligman uses the term eudaimonia, an Aristotelian word meaning "the highest human good" or "human flourishing." As Seligman notes, "Eudaimonia predicts life satisfaction."[228] It means being a part or contributing to something larger than oneself, such as to nature, social

---

[226] Seligman, Martin. (2008, July). Martin Seligman on Positive Psychology [Video file]. Retrieved from http://www.ted.com/talks/martin_seligman_on_the_state_of_psychology.html

[227] Csickzentmihalyi, M. *Flow: the psychology of optimal experience*. Harper and Row: New York, 1990.

[228] Seligman, M (2002). Pleasure, meaning, and eudaimonia. *Authentic Happiness*. Retrieved from http://www.authentichappiness.sas.upenn.edu/newsletter.aspx?id=54.

groups, organizations, movements, or belief systems.

The idea that the meaningful life is more predictive of happiness is evidenced in a study conducted by Veronika Huta of McGill University.[229] Huta followed students and beeped them at random, asking them what they were doing and what their emotional state was. She then quantified the data according to two scales, a hedonic one based on pleasure/comfort/enjoyment and a eudaimonic one based on personal growth/pursuing excellence/contributing to others. Upon conclusion, the study found that "mean eudaimonic activity was significantly predictive of life satisfaction while mean hedonic activity was not." The pursuit of pleasure did not correlate with positive emotion, but the contribution to personal growth or to others did. This information questions the merits of the commonly pursued 'pleasant life' and reveals a part of human nature that is more elevated and complex than commonly thought.

One emotion that exhibits the complexity of human nature was explored by the psychologist Jonathan Haidt of the University of Virginia.[230] He defines it as 'elevation', an emotion of self-transcendence. In his own words, "Elevation is elicited by acts of virtue or moral beauty; it causes warm, open feelings ('dilation?') in the chest; and it motivates people to behave more virtuously themselves."[231] As an evolved trait, elevation is in line with compassion, reciprocal altruism, and the general sense of responsibility to one's loved ones. It highlights a peculiar aspect of human nature: our will to do good for others as it is inspired by the good deeds of others, perhaps hinting that altruism is mechanized by the emotions, and that the emotional upper bound is more sophisticated than most think. This upper bound of emotion is a better place to look for happiness than the less virtuous pleasures of the pleasant life.

---

[229] Huta and Ryan (2010). Pursuing pleasure or virtue: the differential and overlapping well-being benefits of hedonic and eudaimonic motives. *Journal of Happiness Studies* 11: 735-762.

[230] Haidt, J. (2000). "The positive emotion of elevation." *Prevention and Treatment, 3.*

[231] Haidt, J. (2003). "Elevation and the positive psychology of morality." In C. L. M. Keyes & J. Haidt (Eds.) *Flourishing: Positive Psychology and the Life Well-lived.* DC: American Psychological Association. pp. 275-289.

The limitations of the pleasant life on overall well-being and life satisfaction may be due to habituation. Positive psychology has returned to a concept known as 'hedonic adaptation',[232] the tendency for humans to quickly reach a stable level or 'set point' of happiness despite positive or negative changes to their lives.[233] Even drastic changes, such as the sudden inheritance of wealth, may quickly become familiar and lose its effect on overall happiness, returning the individual to their set point regardless of other factors. In the words of psychologist Daniel Gilbert:

> When we have an experience- — hearing a particular sonata, making love with a particular person, watching the sun set from a particular window of a particular room — on successive occasions, we quickly begin to adapt to it, and the experience yields less pleasure each time.[234]

The length of adaptation depends on the degree and nature of the life change; death and unemployment take longer to return to set point than winning a car, for instance. Hedonic adaptation may be a reflection of the chaos of nature. In the wild, our ancestors were subject to constantly changing situations. Therefore, there was no need to evolve a preference for regularity or repetition, revealing why humans naturally crave new experiences. Regardless, hedonic adaptation is one possible explanation for how many seemingly effectual variables to human happiness have been demonstrated to have little or no effect at all. It also points to novelty of experience as a valid strategy for circumventing hedonic adaptation.

Income's role in influencing happiness is popularly misperceived. Most people think that wealth will greatly influence happiness at all levels, which is

---

[232] Brickman and Campbell. "Hedonic Relativism and Planning the Good Society." M.H. Apley, ed., *Adaptation Level Theory: A Symposium*, New York: Academic Press, 1971, pp 287–302.

[233] Lykken, David. *Happiness: What Studies on Twins Show us about Nature, Nurture, and the Happiness Set Point.* Golden Books, 1999.

[234] Gilbert, Daniel. *Stumbling on Happiness.* Vintage, 2007. p 30.

probably why so many strive for riches.[235] While money does significantly influence the well-being of the poor, it does little to influence happiness once basic needs are met.[236] In a paper published in 1974, University of Southern California economist Richard Easterlin noted that in countries with sufficient income to meet their needs, the average reported level of happiness did not vary much, suggesting an upper limit on the ability of money to influence happiness. Similarly, he found that the level of happiness did not increase with rising incomes over the period from 1946 to 1970, further supporting the idea of an upper limit on reported happiness once basic needs are met.

Further supporting the idea that happiness and income is subject to a happiness ceiling is a study by Daniel Kahneman that found self-reported life evaluation to rise continually with income, but not with emotional well-being.[237] At around $75,000 of annual income, respondents reported no additional benefits in emotional state with the rise of income. This supports Easterlin's idea that money contributes very little to happiness once basic needs are met. Every individual has unique needs depending on several factors (family size, possessions, hobbies, etc.). The takeaway message may then be to find an amount that covers basic needs, and to invest further time and resources into developing close personal ties and pursuing elevated life goals.

Another shocking variable that has been shown to be unrelated to happiness is having children. While being a popularly held idea that children bring joy to the lives of parents, this may only be true for married couples.[238] Many studies show that parents of all kinds tend to be worse off in terms of happiness,[239] life satisfaction,[240] marital satisfaction,[241] and mental well-

[235] Aknin, L.; Norton, M.; Dunn, E. (2009). "From wealth to well-being? Money matters, but less than people think." *The Journal of Positive Psychology.* Volume 4 (6): 523–7.

[236] Easterlin, R. (2008). Income and happiness: towards a unified theory. *The Economic Journal.* 11(473): 465-484.

[237] Kahneman D, Deaton A. (2010). "High income improves evaluation of life but not emotional well-being".*Proc. Natl. Acad. Sci. U.S.A.* 107 (38): 16489–93.

[238] Angeles, Luis. (2010). "Children and Life Satisfaction." *Journal of Happiness Studies.* Volume 11 (4) : 523-538.

[239] Alesina et al. (2004). "Inequality and Happiness." *Journal of Public Economics.* Volume 88: 2009-

being[242] compared with non-parents. While this may reflect the difficulty of measuring an abstract, nuanced topic, it may also highlight a misperception about parenting that is rooted in our cultural values. As psychologist Dan Gilbert explains:

> The belief-transmission network of which we are a part cannot operate without a continuously replenished supply of people to do the transmitting, thus the belief that children are a source of happiness becomes a part of our cultural wisdom simply because the opposite belief unravels the fabric of any society that holds it.[243]

Gilbert highlights the role that culture plays in influencing the behavior of a population, a form of evolution vital to modernity. While the science is strong in support of Gilbert's conclusion, it ought to be met with critique. Author and neuroscience journalist Jonah Lehrer, author of bestsellers such as *How We Decide* and *Imagine*, has provided perhaps one of the most cogent rebuttals to the science of parenting and happiness:

> The fact of the matter is that it's much easier to quantify pleasure on a moment-by-moment basis that it is to quantify something as intangible as "meaning" or "love". But just because we can't measure something doesn't mean it isn't important. I actually think one of Bailey's commenters nailed the issue: "I am guessing that if you surveyed marathon runners at various

2042.

[240] Di Tella et al. (2001) "The Macroeconomics of Happiness." 1-40. [PDF] Retrieved via http://parenting.blogs.nytimes.com/2009/04/01/why-does-anyone-have-children.

[241] Twenge et al. (2003). "Parenthood and Marital Satisfaction." *Journal of Marriage and Family.* Volume 65 (3): 574-583.

[242] Clark, Andrew E, and Oswald, Andrew J. (2002). "Well-being in Panels." [PDF] Retrieved via http://parenting.blogs.nytimes.com/2009/04/01/why-does-anyone-have-children.

[243] Gilbert, Daniel. *Stumbling on Happiness.* Random House, 2007.

intervals during the race, they'd complain about how miserable they are. Upon crossing the finish line, they would talk about the overall achievement and how wonderful it was. Same with raising kids."[244]

Child-rearing itself is also a natural part of life due to the evolved mechanisms of lust, attraction, and attachment, which go together in terms of child-rearing.[245] Sexual attraction leads to reproduction, which leads to children. Because people respond on an emotional level to the cues of children, then it is clear that humans have evolved traits that would augment the survivability of the child. Some believe this demonstrates that parenting may be a fundamental need.[246] This would place child-rearing deep into the world of happiness. The overall sense of life fulfillment, pride, and satisfaction of raising kids fits neatly within Seligman's 'meaningful life' as participating in something bigger than oneself, a greater predictor for human happiness than momentary pleasures.

Interestingly, much of human happiness is out of our control. About 50% of our happiness is genetic, passed down as random heritable characteristics like optimism, friendliness, and charm.[247] In one psychologists words,

> ...most people's happiness set-point is above zero, that is, on the happy side of neutral. Nearly 87% of some 2,300 middle-aged twins in our sample rated themselves to be in the upper third in overall, long-term contentment. It seems plausible to suppose that, over the millennia of human evolution, those ancients who

---

[244] Lehrer, Jonah (2008). Happiness and Children. Retreived from the web at http://scienceblogs.com/cortex/2008/02/happiness_and_children.php.

[245] Fisher, Helen (2000). Lust, Attraction, Attachment: Biology and evolution of the three primary emotion systems for mating, reproduction, and parenting. *Journal of Sex Education and Therapy* 25 (1): 96-104.

[246] Bardwick, Judith (1974). Evolution and parenting. *Journal of Social Issues* 30 (4): 39-62.

[247] Lykken, D. and Tellegen, A. (1996). Happiness is a stochastic phenomenon. *Psychological Science* 7 (3).

were grouchy or sad did less well in the struggle for survival and had less luck in the mating game. Our species has become biased toward positive well-being by natural selection.[248]

The social nature of our species certainly does uphold the idea that certain positive traits, such as likeability, would influence one's reproductive success. The genetic component of happiness for human beings today explains how we are programmed to be happy, why we are resilient in the face of tragedy, and why we seek to surround ourselves with others who are happy.

One common, but poorly interpreted, aspect of happiness is the interplay between the mind and body. It presents a burning question: are people healthy because they are happy, or are they happy because they are healthy? Happy people have been found to have more robust immune systems[249] and enjoy greater longevity.[250] So are these findings, and findings like it, due to the happiness, or is the happiness due to the health? Are the two mutually dependent in an upward spiral?

A healthy mind and a healthy body go together because they are intimately interlinked. One salient aspect of the mind-body connection is the enteric nervous system, the human gut. It contains one hundred million neurons, about 90% of the body's serotonin, and about 50% of the body's dopamine. Scientists are currently studying the gut-brain axis as a potential player in psychological disorders, but evidence is rapidly building that the gut (particularly the bacteria within the gut) may play an organ-like role in regulating the nervous system.[251] The implications are that gut bacteria play a role related to serotonin, which associated with overall health[252] and positive

---

[248] Lykken, D. "The Heritability of Happiness." *Harvard Mental Health Letter*. Retrieved from https://www.psych.umn.edu/psylabs/happness/hapindex.htm

[249] Stone et al (1994). Daily events are associated with a secretory immune response to an oral antigen in men. *Health Psychology* 13: 440 – 446.

[250] Danner et al (2001). Positive emotions in early life and longevity: Findings from the nun study. *Journal of Personality and Social Psychology* 80: 804 – 813.

[251] Forsythe et al (2010). Mood and gut feelings. *Brain, Behavior, and Immunity* 24 (1): 9-16.

[252] Young, Simon (2007). How to increase serotonin in the human brain without drugs. *Journal of*

mood.[253] The bacteria in the gut require a proper habitat in order to thrive, which depends on the quality of foods that enter the gut. The vast complexity and importance of the gut exhibits the evolutionary pressure needed to survive (turning food into energy) and matches the layered patterns in nature where ecosystems develop into complex interdependent systems at multiple levels. Thus, eating healthy will ensure proper gut health, influencing proper functioning of the gut, body, and brain. Where does this interdependent cycle start? It starts with food. Normal people sabotage themselves by consuming unnatural foods. The gut-brain axis is a concrete example of the mind-body connection that can be leveraged for better mental health, one that is strengthened by an evolutionary understanding.

Careerism also vies with happiness. Careers force people away from their homes and loved ones. They swallow up a significant amount of time, much of which is inordinately stressful. Careers require indirect time sinks such as commuting, overtime, networking, development, etc. The nature of careerism requires putting one's personal life second to other considerations in order to get ahead, often sacrificing fundamental aspects of human need outside the realm of work or money. As Richard Easterlin writes,

> Because individuals fail to anticipate the extent to which adaptation and social comparison undermine expected utility in the pecuniary domain, they allocate an excessive amount of time to pecuniary goals, and shortchange nonpecuniary ends such as family life and health, reducing their happiness. There is need to devise policies that will yield better-informed individual preferences, and thereby increase individual and societal well-being. [254]

Psychiatry and Neuroscience 32(6): 394–399.

[253] Williams et al (2006). Associations between whole-blood serotonin and positive mood in healthy males. *Biological Psychology* 71(2):171-4.

[254] Easterlin, Richard (2003). Explaining happiness. *National Academy Sciences* 100 (19):11176-11183.

The set point for human happiness is a concept that leads us to question much of the validity surrounding our lives. While careers can be a boon for society, our culture has perhaps taken certain elements of the career too far, expecting marginal benefits in profit and labor maximization at a greater cost to individual and societal well-being.

In terms of time, the workplace has become the most significant arena for adult human social interaction. The average worker spends 45 hours a week working, plus time spent commuting.[255] An increasing number of households contain two working parents, which may decrease the time they can spend together, or with children, or with friends, especially if they're on an unconventional schedule.

The career time sink is troubling because many of the aspects of work are not conducive to forming real relationships. Indeed, much of corporate work culture expressly forbids the development of deep personal ties due to the necessity of professionalism. Professionalism requires that co-workers remain emotionally distant. In this sense, work relationships tend to form less intimately than real relationships, depending on the nature of the work (many careers form relationships that are more intimate), and socializing at work is a far cry from true socializing where individuals form deep intimate bonds based on things like vulnerability, shared secrets, altruism, alliance, loyalty, and shared experience. Sadly, for many people the career becomes the bedrock of social interaction, an ineffective method for satisfying our primal human need for social intimacy and positive social engagement.

One of the fascinating things about the evolution of our species through time was our increasing brain size and intellectuality, thanks largely to new parts of the brain and more sophisticated wiring.[256] Of particular importance to happiness is the pre-frontal cortex, which houses imagination — a key player in our ability to judge scenarios. It's also behind a revelation in

---

[255] From the American Time Use Survey at http://www.bls.gov/tus/

[256] Konopka et al (2012). Human-specific transcriptional networks in the brain. *Neuron* 75 (4): 601-617.

happiness that positive psychologist Dan Gilbert has noted, which is that humans can quite easily synthesize happiness regardless of the scenario; that is, we are capable of creating happiness out of very little, even in the face of tragedy.[257] A loved one dies and, "She's in a better place." Wealth is lost and, "I have no regrets." As imaginative beings we are not only capable, but prone to, synthesizing happiness based on the evolved mechanisms of our brain.

Research has shown that humans are prone to optimism, and that optimism sprouts from specific locations in the brain. Central roles are played by the amygdala and the rostral anterior cingulate cortex.[258] Emotional conflict resolution is also linked to this part of the brain.[259] The evolution of these brain segments makes a few heavy statements about the nature of our species and the emotional state of our culture. First, the fact that these brain regions even exist is a blatant testament to the human animal as one that is naturally exuberant.[260] Most people are hardwired to be optimistic and to deal well with emotional trauma. This implies that emotional trauma was common enough in our evolutionary history to ensure that overcoming it granted a survival advantage. This explains why we deal well with the dark truths of reality (heartbreak, suffering, death) and is certainly a mechanism worth embracing toward the goal of preserving one's own happiness.

Optimism inspires behavior that has rewards but also behavior that has risks. Optimists may be more successful at finding a job,[261] but also more unrealistic about evaluating personal risk,[262] perhaps leading to bad choices. Risk is necessary in order to reap rewards that would enhance survivability,

[257] Gilbert, Daniel (2004). Dan Gilbert asks, Why are we happy? [Video file] Retrieved from http://www.ted.com/talks/dan_gilbert_asks_why_are_we_happy.html

[258] Sharot et al (2007). Neural mechanisms mediatintimisg opm bias. *Nature* 450: 102-105.

[259] Etkin et al (2006). Resolving emotional conflict. *Neuron* 51 (6): 871-882.

[260] For more see: Forencich, Frank. *The Exuberant Animal: the Power of Health, Play, and Joyful Movement.* AuthorHouse, 2006.

[261] Kaniel et al (2010). The importance of being an optimist. *National Bureau of Economic Research.* Working paper no. 16328.

[262] Neil D. Weinstein and William M. Klein, (1996). Unrealistic Optimism: Present and Future. *Journal of Social and Clinical Psychology* 15(1): pp. 1-8.

but often the mechanisms that spur risk-taking (in part, optimism) would parallel bad choices as well, such as not putting on sunblock or not wearing a seatbelt. It becomes important then to consciously identify where risks are warranted and where they are not, lest allow one's basic nature to get the better of them.

Lastly, I'd like to point out the interconnectedness of everything. The insight that happiness starts with food and ends with selflessness is a testament to all the topics of this book, all of them relevant to a discussion about happiness. The chapters before this one, and the chapters that follow, only further refine what we mean by this loaded word.

Strategies for Happiness

Expand, identify, and fulfill basic needs. Not only should we look at health as a central component of happiness, but other needs too: our intimate relationships, our place within a close group of friends and/or a community of people, the respect we give and receive, etc. Maslow's hierarchy is a great reference point.

Build close circles of quality friends, family, and lovers. The people in life are far more important than most realize. More on this in Chapter 8 when we unravel the mysteries of love and human sexuality.

Garner and embrace new experiences. Novelty is the spice of life, and monotony will deaden your zest for it. Nassim Taleb once said, "If you know, in the morning, what your day looks like with any precision, you are a little bit dead — the more precision, the more dead."

Earn the highest emotions. Love, elevation, glory, eudaimonia. Victory is a real emotion but you can only feel it if you've won big. There are things more profound than the hedonic pleasures and they should be on your radar, too. They are characterized by selflessness and virtue. More on this in Chapter 9.

Find 'flow' wherever and whenever possible. This means absorbing yourself in work and play to the degree that 'time flies'. It means relishing the momentary joys, pleasures, and social interactions of life as they occur. The moments of life demand your attention — allow them to engage you. Mindfulness meditation may help.

Seek meaning in the grand scheme. This means placing your skills and passions within a broader context of importance, such as contributing to a movement, following passions, devoting oneself to others, or seeking a higher path of wisdom. It's not exactly what you end up choosing, but what it means to you that is important.

"There is new life in the soil for every man. There is healing in the trees for tired minds and for our overburdened spirits, there is strength in the hills, if only we will lift up our eyes. Remember that nature is your great restorer."

Calvin Coolidge

Number 30

"Forget not that the earth delights to feel your bare feet and the winds long to play with your hair."

Kahlil Gibran

Lebanese-American poet

CHAPTER 7

THE RESTORATIVE ASPECTS OF NATURE

The first photosynthesis is believed to have evolved out of the bacteria of early Earth approximately 3.5 billion years ago.[263] It was a turning point for the evolution of life on Earth, harnessing a powerful new way to derive energy from sunlight. Photosynthesis is a process that speaks volumes about the potential for life to take advantage of the resources available to it, and for the fascinating nature by which life on Earth is interconnected beyond the worldly ecology to a cosmological one — all the way to a star 100 million miles away.

Plants need the sun, but so do human beings. In fact, we are more intimately reliant on the sun than many realize. Not only do we take advantage of the natural ecologies that develop thanks to the sun's energy, but our health also relies on the sunlight that hits our skin, light that originates from a thermonuclear reaction at the sun's core. We need sunlight to regulate melatonin, to manufacture vitamin D, and perhaps even to ensure our cardiovascular health.[264] These processes point to the intimate

---

[263] Blankenship, Robert (2010). Early Evolution of Photosynthesis. *Plant Physiology* 154 (2): 434-438.

[264] Feelisch et al (2010). Is sunlight good for our heart? *European Heart Journal* 31 (9): 1041-1045.

interconnectivity of nature and our place within it. It represents a definitive, concrete example of how exposure to nature has a positive effect on our bodies, something that should be predictable given what we know about evolution.

It is predictable from an evolutionary perspective that the sun would confer health benefits. We evolved under the sun, after all. Sunlight on our skin is as warranted as the air in our lungs and the blood in our veins. Yet a lot of old science (and some bad science) led to the rise of flawed conventional wisdoms about the sun's harm, particularly that well-known wisdom: the sun causes cancer. *The sun causes cancer?* To understand our place in nature is to understand that statements like these are absurd. *Does the air cause asthma?* More reasonable statements must take a measured approach: excess sun exposure may contribute to the development of cancer in immunodeficient people. There is a canyon of meaning between these two statements. One falsely paints us into a corner, pegged against nature; the other describes a complex and mysterious biological and historical phenomenon.

Recently, however, medical establishments have toned down their warnings about sun exposure. A 2007 study concludes,

> These data, together with those for internal cancers and the beneficial effects of an optimal vitamin D status, indicate that increased sun exposure may lead to improved cancer prognosis and, possibly, give more positive than adverse health effects.[265]

As scientific methodologies improve and our conclusions are sharpened, it is most effective to fit our findings within a matrix of understanding. To embed that information somewhere that makes sense. Evolution is that matrix. It is the overarching theme of human well-being that ties these ideas together. But the nature connection goes much deeper than sunlight. Evolution has clues as to our place in nature not only in terms of the biological necessities that

---

[265] Moan et al (2007) Addressing the health benefits and risks, involving Vitamin D or skin cancer, of increased sun exposure. *PNAS* 105 (2): 668-673.

govern our interaction with the environment, such as in sun exposure, but also in the psychological harmony of our day-to-day lives.

For most of 2011, the city of Lancaster, California operated over seventy loudspeakers throughout its town. But instead of music, it played subtle synth tones and birdsong for five hours each day. According to its mayor, the birdsong was to thank for a 15% drop in petty crime and 6% drop in serious crime.[266] As the rationale goes: the birdsong made people feel more pleasant, and pleasant people simply commit less crime. Could there be something more to this phenomenon?

Julian Treasure is a sound health expert out of London, England, where he consults businesses on how to use the science of sound to their advantage. In a TED Talk about the importance of sound to health, he highlights that many of the sounds that are beneficial to the human mind are the ones found in nature, naming wind, water, and birdsong as positive stochastic events throughout human evolution.[267] Thus, the reduction in crime in Lancaster, California may very well have been due to the elevated mood of its population.

The evolutionary perspective regarding the positive sounds of nature points to many things commonly regarded as pleasing, such as children at play or the calls of animals. But how would enjoying nature present an evolutionary advantage? One explanation may be that many of these sounds are simply indicative of a healthy ecology where food would be easier to procure. Indeed, any signs of life would do. Therefore, humans are naturally predisposed to look favorably at cues of life that represent a more promising environment for survival.

So what else indicates a healthy ecology, and does that play into our hard-wired preferences for nature? One major contributing factor to a layered ecology of animals is a layered ecology of plants. Since most plants are green due to their chlorophyll content, then it's reasonable to predict from an

---

[266] Cooke, Sonia (Jan 2012). California town wards off crime with birdsong. *Time Magazine*.

[267] Treasure, J (2010). Julian Treasure: Shh! Sound health in 8 steps. [Video file] Retrieved from http://www.ted.com/talks/julian_treasure_shh_sound_health_in_8_steps.html.

evolutionary perspective that green may also contribute positively to the mental and physical health of the individual. Studies support that green has a relaxing, comforting effect on people due to its resemblance of nature,[268] thus aiding their mental and physical health through stress relief.

So what about silence? As the saying goes, "Silence is golden." But health benefits of total silence might not seem to fit an evolutionary perspective. Total silence in nature would imply desolation, solitude, and the absence of life. Thus, how can we reconcile the idea that silence may be health-promoting, as Julian Treasure, the sound health expert, says it will, if silence does not fit an evolutionary perspective?

The answer may lie in the discord between how we evolved and the modern lives we live. Millions of people live in environments full of noise that detract from our health. Things like construction, traffic, and aircraft impact public health and personal psyche negatively. Studies have found that noise increases wakefulness due to cortisol (stress hormone) release,[269] which leads to sleep deprivation.[270] Noise increases blood pressure in children,[271] and daytime noise has been demonstrated to impair children's cognitive performance at school.[272] Noise is also related to the development of heart disease.[273] Thus, it may be the lack of noise that leads to benefits, rather than the silence itself. On the other hand, silence can also be an environment conducive to focus and meditation, an environment free from distraction and negative sound inputs. In this way, seeking silence in certain situations may be an advantage to focus, productivity, and relaxation. Some have gone so far as

---

[268] Epps, Helen and Kaya, Naz (2004). Relationship between color and emotion: a study of college students. *College Student Journal* 38 (3).

[269] Basner et al (2010). Effects of aircraft noise on sleep. *Sleep and Noise* 12 (47): 95-109.

[270] Tetreault et al (2012). Review of aircraft noise on sleep disturbance in adults. *Sleep and Noise* 14(57): 58-67.

[271] Belojevic et al (2011). Cardiovascular effects of environmental noise: research in Serbia. *Sleep and Noise* 13 (52): 217-220.

[272] Stansfield et al (2010). Nighttime aircraft exposure and children's cognitive performance at school. *Sleep and Noise* 12 (49): 255-262

[273] Ndrepepa et al (2011). Relationship between road traffic noise and cardiovascular disease: a meta-analysis. *Sleep and Noise* 13(52): 251-259.

to tout the benefits of sensory deprivation tanks. Hey, whatever works.

Evolution, Music, and Healing

In contrast to the annoyance of noise, have you ever considered why you so viscerally enjoy music? It turns out that music may be a positive sound that exists as part of our evolutionary heritage. Charles Darwin once said:

> ...if I had to live my life again, I would have made a rule to read some poetry and listen to some music at least once every week; for perhaps the parts of my brain now atrophied would thus have been kept active through use. The loss of these tastes is a loss of happiness, and may possibly be injurious to the intellect, and more probably to the moral character, by enfeebling the emotional part of our nature.[274]

In 2001, researchers from the Washington University School of Medicine found that heightened enjoyment of music was related to the brain's reward center. In the researchers' own words,

> These brain structures are known to be active in response to other euphoria-inducing stimuli, such as food, sex, and drugs of abuse. This finding links music with biologically relevant, survival-related stimuli via their common recruitment of brain circuitry involved in pleasure and reward.[275]

This points to music as having some of the driving elements of addiction. This may seem scary, but I assure you that there are not many negative outcomes

---

[274] Darwin, Charles. *The Descent of Man*. 1897.

[275] Blood and Zattore (2001). Intensely pleasurable responses to music correlate with brain regions implicated in reward and emotion. *National Academy of Sciences* 98 (20): 11818-11823.

associated with abusing music. While sad or aggressive music can adversely affect one's mood, choosing positive music about love or community, for example, will likewise have a positive psychological impact.[276]

The therapeutic benefits of music are clearly demonstrated in patients with degenerative disease or trauma. In patients with Parkinson's, music has been shown to increase motor performance[277] and improve the precision and coordination of arm and hand movements.[278] In stroke patients, exposure to music improves cognition, increases motivation and awareness, and generally bolsters positive mood.[279] [280] If there are tangible benefits in music therapy for patients, wouldn't those benefits also apply to normal people? While it may seem silly or obvious to suggest that music can be beneficial for normal people, the idea is just one more drop in the bucket that reveals how our biology and psychology can be leveraged to our advantage through modern means, all thanks to evolution.

There is a rich world of evolutionary hypotheses surrounding music. Most consider music itself to be a communication system that evolved just like language.[281] Some of the indications of this are intriguing. In particular, enjoyable music has been shown to affect the social part of the brain, where we form social concepts,[282] and manage mutual cooperative advantage

---

[276] Treasure, J (2010). Julian Treasure: Shh! Sound health in 8 steps. [Video file] Retrieved from http://www.ted.com/talks/julian_treasure_shh_sound_health_in_8_steps.html.

[277] Frazzita et al (2009). Rehabilitation treatment of gait in patients with Parkinson's disease with freezing: a comparison between two physical therapy protocols using visual and auditory cues with or without treadmill training. *Movement Disorders* 24: 1139-43.

[278] Sacrey et al (2009). Music attenuates excessive visual guidance of skilled reaching in advanced but not mild Parkinson's disease. *PLoS ONE* 4(8): e6841.

[279] Sarkarmo et al (2008). Music listening enhances cognitive recovery and mood after middle cerebral artery stroke. *Brain* 131: 866-76.

[280] Forsblum et al (2009). Therapeutic role of music listening in stroke rehabilitation. In: *The Neurosciences and Music III - Disorders and Plasticity, Annal of the New York Academy of Science* 1169: 426-430.

[281] Harvey, Alan (2011). "Evolution, Music, and Neurotherapy" in *Pragmatic Evolution* [Ed. Aldo Poiani]. Cambridge University Press, 2012.

[282] Zahn et al (2007). Social concepts are represented in the superior anterior temporal cortex. Proceeding so the National Academy of Sciences 104: 6430-5.

(reciprocal altruism).[283] Thus, music is implicated as a medium through which humans collectively experience and express emotions, which provides an evolutionary advantage to the group via group cohesion and cooperation.[284] So the next time you feel particularly moved by a song, you'll see just how deeply and intricately music affects our consciousness.

The Nature Connection

The nature connection has seen a good deal of exploration by scientists, and it's a hypothesis that makes perfect sense in terms of evolution. After all, our ancestors spent all of their time in the wild. One of the first to popularly explore this topic was Edward O. Wilson in 1984, who questioned the nearly universal human obsession with other life forms. In his own words,

> The object of the reflection can be summarized by a single word, biophilia, which I will be so bold as to define as the innate tendency to focus on life and lifelike processes...From infancy we concentrate happily on ourselves and other organisms. We learn to distinguish life from the inanimate and move toward it like moths to a porchlight. Novelty and diversity are particularly esteemed; the mere mention of the word extraterrestrial evokes reveries about still unexplored life, replacing the old and once potent exotic that drew earlier generations to remote islands and jungled interiors...I will make the case that to explore and affiliate with life is a deep and complicated process in mental development. To an extent still undervalued in philosophy and religion, our existence depends on this propensity, our spirit is

---

[283] Rilling et al (2008). The neurobiology of social decision-making. *Current Opinions in Neurobiology* 18: 159-65.

[284] Harvey, Alan (2011). "Evolution, Music, and Neurotherapy" in *Pragmatic Evolution* [Ed. Aldo Poiani]. Cambridge University Press, 2012.

woven from it, hope rises on its currents.[285]

He defines biophilia as an "innate tendency" that our "existence depends on." Indeed, from an evolutionary perspective, biophilia may simply underlie how survival requires participating with other life forms. Hunting, foraging, reading weather, evaluating threat, and finding water are all pivotal parts of life in the wild that involve the interaction with other life forms or lifelike processes. This itself may demonstrate the evolved trait of biophilia — one that is simply required in order for life to survive.

Biophilia highlights an additional way that modernity vies with the evolutionary history of humans. One researcher interprets biophilia as out of line with human evolution in the modern context:

> Wilson's biophilia hypothesis, which suggests that because humans evolved in natural environments and have lived separate from nature only relatively recently in their evolutionary history, people possess an innate need to affiliate with other living things...Nature can also be a source of happiness. Humans evolved in natural environments and still seem to thrive in them...Modern lifestyles, however, may erode people's connection with nature, leaving them unaware of nature's potential benefits. By limiting their contact with nature, people fail to maximize the advantages it offers for cognition and well-being.[286]

The rise of civilization has led many away from nature. For some, the degree to which they have lost touch may leave them wanting subconsciously. This may carry implications for the development and maintenance of physical and mental health for people who find themselves far removed from the

---

[285] Wilson, E.O. *Biophilia*. Harvard University Press, 1984.

[286] Nisbet and Zelenski (2011). Understanding Nearby Nature: Affective forecasting features obscure the happy path to sustainability. *Psychological Science* 22 (9): 1101-1106.

restorative aspects of nature.

Exposure to nature may also have health benefits. Not only have observational population studies found that exposure to nature can decrease mortality significantly, but also that contact with nature can restore attention, augment creativity,[287] improve concentration in children with ADHD, speed recovery from illness, and reduce stress.[288] These findings are in line with an evolutionary perspective when they highlight the detriment that modern living may add to one's psychological and physiological well-being, not to mention the benefits that exposure to nature may preclude.

Nature also has the ability to augment our happiness and increase our desire to do good by the environment. Scientists measure this on a scale called nature relatedness — the affective, cognitive, and experiential connection to nature — and it is positively associated with well-being. In fact, an affective connection to nature also leads to sustainable behavior in regard to the environment.[289] For children, having animals as pets may also fuel this connection to the environment.[290] By creating an avenue for a modern child to form a relationship with another species, pets may be a potent replacement for the ancient necessity to engage other species simply as a matter of survival, a behavior unnecessary in modern life. Since modern life can disconnect us from nature then fostering the nature connection however possible may prove beneficial.

Ultimately, we are animals that seek connection to each other and to nature. We are fascinated by the mysticism of lightning bolts. We adore observing kittens at play. We cherish the music of rushing streams and rivers. There is something to be said about the loss of these things from modern life

---

[287] Atchley RA, Strayer DL, Atchley P (2012) Creativity in the Wild: Improving Creative Reasoning through Immersion in Natural Settings. *PLoS ONE* 7(12): e51474.

[288] Mitchell and Popham (2008). Effect of exposure to natural environment on health inequalities: an observational population study. *The Lancet* 372 (9650): 1655-1660.

[289] Nisbet et al (2011). Happiness is in our nature: exploring nature relatedness as a contributor to our subjective well-being. *Journal of Happiness Studies* 12 (2): 303-322.

[290] Kahn and Kellert. *Children and Nature: Psychological, Sociocultural, and Evolutionary Investigations.* MIT Press, 2002.

that used to fulfill an ancient part of our psyche. Perhaps it is up to us to reclaim this part of our nature and set our own standards as to how much we need.

"A touch of nature makes the whole world kin."

Shakespeare, quill enthusiast

Strategies in Nature Connection

Get adequate sunlight. There are myriad benefits to health and beauty by consistently getting a little sun on as much skin as possible.

Make a habit of nature. It doesn't have to be the backcountry of Alaska. There are many parks and places that resemble the sights and sounds of the wild. Simply spending time at the city park or getting a pet may be a worthy compromise.

Practice awareness of sounds. Noise might affect your mood more than you realize. There are simple cures for noise, like earplugs or headphones. Or, if you want to get really crazy, try out a sensory deprivation tank.

Leverage the power of positive music. There is a time and place for sad songs or intense, rowdy music, but these may not necessarily put us at ease. Try to find something you like that promotes positive feelings and contains positive messages.

On the Ethics of Meat-Eating

Let's get deep for a moment. Let's zoom out of the sandbox of earthly evolution that we have buried our heads in and think of the entire universe. Our cold, dark, dead universe. Lifeless matter afloat in space. Starry driftwood as far as the eye can see. Everywhere but here on Earth, so far as we know, because we are lucky. We are very, very lucky.

When Cormac McCarthy, arguably the greatest American writer alive, took the topic of the universe into his skilled hands in order to craft a literary passage in one of his stories, he wrote,

> He walked out in the gray light and stood and he saw for a brief moment the absolute truth of the world. The cold relentless circling of the intestate earth. Darkness implacable. The blind dogs of the sun in their running. The crushing black vacuum of the universe. And somewhere two hunted animals trembling like ground-foxes in their cover. Borrowed time and borrowed world and borrowed eyes with which to sorrow it.[291]

I don't intend to recall another dark truth about the world; I intend to drive the reality of nature into your understanding.

Life is precious. That's something that everyone can agree on. But why is life precious? Is it precious for its hallowed nature? A mysterious, empyreal ingredient of mother Earth? Is it precious due to some abstract inclination, an inviolable sentiment?

---

[291] McCarthy, Cormac. *The Road.* Vintage, 2007.

Life is precious because it's a miracle, a rare natural phenomenon that, as far as we know from a scientific perspective, arose out of the chaos of nature. The dead elements of life swam about the Earth for an eternity until one day they arranged in just the right way, in just the right environment, that the rudiments of life were forged. Then cells. Then organisms. Then animals. And brains. And consciousness. And emotion. And then, finally, true intelligence. That is why life is precious, because out of stardust, the miracle of life sprang, and developed into dynamic, beautiful, interconnected ecosystems that waxed and waned and vanished and flourished over the millennia, undergoing extinctions and leaps, until finally arriving where we are now. It's an unlikely journey that has brought us here. It's one that is sacred and delicate and wonderful.

Of all the life forms that descended from the universal common ancestor, some are more precious than others. Some have achieved consciousness, others have not. Some have achieved emotion, others have not. And only one species on our planet has achieved true intelligence, so far as we know in the universe, leaps and bounds ahead of any other species, more than is even required by the environment for survival, a misstep in the evolutionary process, a lucky strike in the lottery of natural law. In this way, some forms of life are objectively more miraculous than others. Bacteria is ultimately less precious than, say, an animal. A worm is less precious than, say, a rat. A rat is less precious than, say, an eagle (they achieved flight, after all). And at the very top of this totem pole, I would place humans, as most would, because we have achieved all that other species have and more. We are intelligent, compassionate, moral, long-lived, and industrious. We are the world's hope, the world's threat. For all intents and purposes, we are gods walking the earth. Imperfect, often irrational gods with the potential to surpass even our own potential.

In 2012, *The New York Times* held a contest for its readers, who were asked to submit essays about the ethics of meat-eating. The essays were reviewed by a panel of judges that included big names like Mark Bittman, Jonathan Safran Foer, Michael Pollan, Andrew Light, and Peter Singer. It was meant to incite and explore the morality of killing and eating animals. The winning essay was written by a former vegan and vegetarian who began eating meat after studying ecology at advanced levels. He wrote:

> For me, eating meat is ethical when one does three things. First, you accept the biological reality that death begets life on this planet and that all life (including us!) is really just solar energy temporarily stored in an impermanent form. Second, you combine this realization with that cherished human trait of compassion and choose ethically raised food, vegetable, grain and/or meat. And third, you give thanks.[292]

His essay on the subject is short and simple. It acknowledges the harsh realities of the world, its ecologies based on predation, where the circle of life is brutal and murderous, yet at the same time wondrous and humbling.

But I find this conclusion lacking, because I do not believe in the black and white of ethical behavior. The entire discussion is oversimplified from the outset: is it ethical, or not ethical? I am a strategist, an optimist, and I believe that ethics are scalable, that certain choices are more ethical than others. And I believe that ethical choices can be optimized.

---

[292] Bost, Jay (2012). The Ethicist Contest Winner: Give Thanks for Meat. *New York Times*. [Web file] Retrieved from http://www.nytimes.com/2012/05/06/magazine/the-ethicist-contest-winner-give-thanks-for-meat.html

To choose meat-eating is to participate in a mutually beneficial ecological relationship. However, it is a novel relationship, historically, because by choosing to eat naturally raised animals we give those animals the gift of life. It is life in addition to and apart from most life in the wild. Indeed, choosing naturally raised animals increases the net quantity of our cherished animals in the world, and the net life on this planet. After all, farm animals are born to be eaten, and would never see the light of day otherwise.

With the goal of maximizing the quantity of precious life forms, eating animals that were raised on farms today is wholly different than hunting animals in the wild. Our ancestors who hunted in the wild played a natural role in the ecology as apex predators, a role they sometimes overplayed. Though for them, the animals they chose were out of necessity, based on survival.

Today, we have the opportunity to hunt overpopulated species and to choose animals that are born outside the world of the wild, animals born into the comforts of the farm, where they are mostly protected from the hardships of the wild. In the wild, animals are killed viciously, often eaten alive. On farms, they are more safe, more fed, and more happy than they would be in the wild, and their deaths are comparatively merciful. Just like you and I prefer the comforts of civilization, so would the domesticated animal prefer the comforts of the farm. And on farms, we control the animal population based on demand. Therefore, the more we eat naturally raised meat, the more happy animals get to live out their lives.

For this simple reason, it is not only ethical — it is *more* ethical — to eat animals than to eat plants, because animals are more precious life forms than plants. Ironically, this also happens to be a premise within some arguments for vegetarianism/veganism, which avoid eating animals, because sentience and consciousness grants animals the right to life. If all life forms were equal, then it wouldn't matter which ones we ate; plants and animals would be fair game. We instinctively rank conscious beings higher, as we should. Hence, the vegetarian premise is valid, but the course of its logic is not. (The vegan/vegetarian conclusion of avoiding conventionally-raised and industrialized meats, however, is a perfectly valid notion that I uphold passionately as well. In fact, none of my arguments apply to this industrial model. Much more on this in the final chapter about sustainability.)

Choosing vegetarianism/veganism is to choose to lower the demand for ethically raised meat. Less demand for meat means less happy animals running around on farmland. Therefore, to not eat animals is to abort them. That's even more blood on your hands, especially in light of the fact that choosing to eat them is to give these animals the gift of life. It's one or the other, and the higher path is clear.

An inevitable death does not cancel the value, meaning, and beauty of life. Wouldn't you choose life if it meant one day you would die? Isn't that the bargain with God you and I have made already?

It is optimal, ethically, to deliberately promote the proliferation of precious, complex forms of life through one's dietary choices, and to ensure that those animals live well during their lives.

We operate within an intimate context of nature, embedded in a world that interacts delicately and broadly at all layers. These layers depend on one another, giving and taking in a complex, mutually beneficial cycle, all for the sake of sustaining the most precious and sacred manifestation of our dead universe: the gift of life.

The Evolution of Dogs

Many people love pets. They bring joy to the household, and fill our lives with love, life, and energy, playing roles as additional characters in the story of our lives. The connection to them is real and fulfilling. So it may come as a surprise that many people don't really understand where dogs come from and why we love them so much. Like many things, it's only evolution that explains this fully.

Consider that there are no poodles in the wild. There are no Chihuahuas in the deserts of Mexico, nor German shepherds in the woodlands of Bavaria. The diverse and unique breeds of canines that exist today are simply descendants of the wild animals that humans domesticated long ago. In fact, all dogs descend probably from grey wolves or perhaps from wild dogs,[293] having evolved over thousands of years of human domestication and selective breeding. They are themselves subject to a mechanism of evolution called 'artificial selection'. They were bred for certain traits, such as hunting skills, trainability, aesthetics, and friendliness. However, these traits were not selected for by nature; instead, they were selected for by breeders, by humans. All domesticated dogs today are therefore representative of a simple mechanism of evolution, the selection of traits. Artificial selection has proven to be a more potent form of evolution than natural selection, which is slowed by the random forces of nature. Human hands can select genetic traits with more precision than nature can, singularly guiding a species toward certain ends.

How exactly dogs were domesticated is under debate. The first solid evidence of domestication is a burial site, only about 14,000 years old,[294] but some believe that ancient humans adopted wolf pups to some degree as far back as 135,000 years ago.[295] Pups that were less aggressive were selected for breeding by the humans caring for them.

---

[293] Druzhkovka et al (2013). Ancient DNA analysis affirms the canid from Altai as primitive dog. *PLoS ONE* 8(3): e57754.

[294] Udell and Wynne (2008). A review of domestic dogs' (canis familiaris) human-like behaviors: Or why behavioral analysts should stop worrying and love their dogs. Journal of the Experimental Analysis of Behavior 89(2): 247–261.

[295] Vilà et al (1997). Multiple and ancient origins of the domestic dog. *Science* 276 (5319):1687-9.
295

Others argue that wolves domesticated themselves slowly by learning to feed near humans. It makes sense that wolves would take advantage of the scavenging opportunities near human encampments and that eventually those dogs would rely more and more on humans, leading to their full domestication. Every domesticated dog species today relies on humans for survival. Even semi-wild ones that scavenge villages still require proximity to humans in order to survive.

This makes sense of a lot of dog behavior, does it not? It is only in this context that we can understand why dogs bark at other dogs so aggressively. Why they mark their territory. Why they love their 'wolfpack' so dearly. We have evolution to thank for these friendly canines. They represent a beautiful manifestation of human ingenuity when the human hand is applied to nature. And they are one more thing that makes sense in the light of evolution.

Why do the Swedish tan better than the British, despite being at a higher latitude?

Evolution predicts that skin color is simply an adaptation to varying levels of light. Humans need to synthesize vitamin D from the sun's UVB rays, and at higher latitudes, these rays are increasingly weakened. However, many Swedish people retain the genetic ability to bronze naturally while most British do not. The answer to this puzzle lies in the environment. In Sweden, there is snow for much of the year. In the United Kingdom, there is a significant amount of fog, but little snow. Snow reflects the sun's rays back up off the surface of the ground while fog diminishes the sun's rays before they reach the ground. In Sweden's environment, people are actually doubly exposed to sunlight as the rays come down and then are reflected up off the ground. Hence, the Swedish retain a higher level of exposure than the British, despite the high latitude and the cold-weather clothing. The fog will cut UVB significantly, which increases the skin's need, and in turn human skin adapts by whitening. In this way, the most pale skin will be found in those whose direct ancestors hail from an environment with lowest levels of light, not simply the ones closest to Earth's poles.

Why Not Just Go Back to the Wild?

Taking evolutionary interpretation to its logical conclusion, some will inevitably reach this question. I'll answer it bluntly. Desmond Morris, who literally made a zoological study of humans, once said about civilization, "It's not a concrete jungle. It's a human zoo." But wild animals in captivity are a false analogy to humans in society. We are not wild animals in cages. We are domesticated animals walking padded floors with padded shoes, eating pet food from tin cans and plastic bags. We get too cold and too hot and can't go long without eating. We need a soft mattress and a flashlight in the night. Like pets, we are a domesticated species, layers and layers removed from our natural surroundings, unfit for the rigor of nature on the genetic level. Richard Manning said in an interview, "[If] hunter-gatherers watched behavior of people in our society, they would think we were crazy for the way we behave, because we are." We are the grazing cattle, safely behind barb wire fences, holding the keys to our own feedlots, giving a significant portion of our lives to those more powerful through the exploitation of labor, another gift of evolution in the form of economic efficiency. We are insane farm animals, comfortably consuming and regurgitating what has become of human culture. Surely, it tastes good. But it's not all good for us, and we know deep down that it's not what we're supposed to be doing.

Chris McCandless probably knew this in his heart when he famously went back into the wild by himself. If you've ever read the book by Jon Krakauer or seen the movie, *Into the Wild*, directed by

Sean Penn, then you know he died at the end. That's not a spoiler, that's a fact. You, nor I, nor Bear Grylls can survive in the wild alone at any length without modern technology. In the movie, McCandless's last revelation is that happiness is meant to be shared with others. That's true, too, because you can't survive alone.

Most people are invested in the reality they've inherited. Most are not strong enough to radically change the way they live their lives, and who can blame them? Would you send a poodle back into the wild? Everyone who reads this book is going to make their own compromises and that's fine. All we can do is look back while carving out a new future going forward. This is the promise of evolutionary interpretation.

"Men are from Mars, women are from Venus."

John Gray

bestselling relationship author

"Men are from Africa, women are from Africa."

Christopher Ryan

bestselling human sexuality author

CHAPTER 8

THE INTERSECTIONS OF SEX, ATTRACTION, BEAUTY, LOVE, AND TRIBE

You probably never thought about why humans have sex. Not why people choose to have sex with each other, but why human beings even have sex to begin with. There is great fascination as to how, when, where, and who is having sex, even in popular media and as part of daily gossip. But *why* just seems to evade us.

As it turns out, almost every animal on Earth replicates its genes through male-female reproduction. There are exceptions, such as in jellyfish, but the vast majority of animals on Earth have found male-female reproduction to efficiently fill the evolutionary need to carry on genes. This is due to the fact that male-female pairs have an evolutionary advantage over all other forms of reproduction. Had a third 'sex' appeared in addition to males and females, and had that third sex gleaned an evolutionary advantage from a three-sex environment, then there would be a third sex here with us today, and humans would have another gender to complain about. However, for most animals, the two-sex pair is where we stand, all due to the efficient advantage of two-sex reproduction.

The driving force of reproduction is sexual attraction. It is one of the most potent of all traits, rooted deeply into the reward system of our brains, right along with food. As such, sex is a primal human need for survival (that is, the survival of one's genetic material). The evolutionary advantage of sex drive makes perfect sense: high levels of sex drive leads to more sex, which leads to the proliferation of genes through reproduction.

For this reason, human beings today seek out sex, as do all animals in the animal kingdom, because sex itself is a fundamental requirement of evolution — one necessary for the very existence of a species. Without it, life cannot go on. Consider the panda, which is at risk of extinction, and at the same time, is commonly known to be lacking in the libido department. Panda bears are reluctant to mate, which presents a huge problem in preventing their extinction. The example of the panda bear highlights how attraction is a driving element of reproduction, which in turn drives adaptation. It is crucially important from an evolutionary perspective. Our evolved mechanisms of love can even outweigh our need to survive. In the words of the prominent sexologist Helen Fisher, "People live for love. They kill for love. They die for love. They have songs, poems, novels, sculptures, paintings, myths, legends. It's one of the most powerful brain systems on Earth for both great joy and great sorrow."

Human Kink

Many animals have to wait for a small window of time to open for breeding. Still others engage in aggressive behavior, leading to fighting or taking mates forcibly. Most animals last merely seconds, and simply insert their penis statically until ejaculation. Humans display some interesting differences. Compared to other animals, humans were blessed by the evolutionary process, because sex for us is, in many ways, just better.

Consider the human penis, which is the largest out of all the primates. It's bigger both relative to body size and in absolute terms. That's right, boys, in all probability, you have a bigger penis than a gorilla. While the reasons behind the relatively large human penis are still under debate, many things seem to make sense. Longer penises eject sperm closer to the egg, therefore perhaps increasing reproductive odds. Penises are also unconcealed in nature and rely on basic physiology to function, so our female ancestors may have seen the penis as a marker for fertility and, therefore, suitability in mate choice. But above all the human penis got big because it was important. The many evolutionary interpretations of penis size all point to human sexuality taking a unique direction distinct from our hominid cousins. But it's not only the penis that received an evolutionary blessing. So did the vagina.

Human females retain the ability to intensely enjoy the sensory feedback of sex due to the relatively large amount of nerve endings in and around the vagina, as especially located in the clitoris. In fact, the clitoris has nearly twice the nerve endings of the penis.[296] Many females today are capable of achieving orgasm despite the fact that orgasm is unnecessary to become pregnant, and many females are capable of achieving orgasm frequently. The female orgasm may have evolved not as a biological necessity for reproduction per se, but as a driving factor leading to the pursuit of sex. Since orgasm would incentivize females to have more sex than otherwise, it may alter female sexual behavior enough to increase odds of reproduction.[297] Some even argue that the female orgasm is vestigial, stemming from the male's genome much like men inherit nipples from the female's genome. This topic remains an unsolved mystery. There may be multiple evolutionary pressures at work, but humans are lucky to have this adaptation. Obviously.

Humans are also capable of frequent sexual intercourse. Men and women are capable of sex multiple times per day, and even of taking multiple partners in a short time frame. There is no seasonal breeding window as there is in other animals, enabling us to have children throughout the year. The human brain may have been a factor leading to the evolution of year-long reproduction, since our use of tools, shelter, and clothing were protective against infant mortality during the challenging environment of prehistory.

Humans have sex for reasons other than procreation. In fact, clinical

---

[296] Carroll, J. *Sexuality Now: Embracing Diversity.* Cengage, 2012. pp 110-111, 152.

[297] Morris, Desmond. *The Naked Ape.* Delta, 1969. pp 79-80.

psychologist Cindy Meston and evolutionary psychologist David Buss found that women have sex for 237 reasons ranging from the altruistic to the evil.[298] The vast complexity of human sexuality is a testament to human emotion, human motivation, and human psychobiology. We are, in fact, the result of the chaos of the evolutionary environment, one where the give and take of survival advantage and reproductive fitness left us with a vast array of compromising traits.

The Game of Lust

There are songs and movies about love. There are sonnets and stories. There are celebrations and books and websites. It is clear that love is a force to be reckoned with. Our species is crazy about love. It may be the most potent cascade of biochemicals that we own. Understanding attraction, lust, and love, therefore, is very important to the quality of one's life.

The words "lust" and "attraction" are among many nebulous words we use to describe human longing. They attempt to encapsulate not only the instinct of physical sexual attraction, but also the social and emotional yearning for the affection of others, again highlighting that human mating systems are governed by biological, psychological, and social parameters.

As the standard theory goes, the androgen and estrogen hormones govern sex drive in both males and females, with men having elevated sex drive, relatively, thanks to significantly higher levels of testosterone. Tradition teaches us that this makes men the agents of mate selection, as they are the ones who are more biologically compelled to give chase, make moves, and push the envelope. But there is more to this story.

Women are not passive deciders, but active participants in mate selection. They hunt, too, for they have significant sex drive, and exhibit many interesting behaviors regarding the agency of mate selection. Most obviously, women exert great effort to attract attention. Grooming, face and body paint

---

[298] Meston and Buss. *Why Women Have Sex*. Times, 2009

(make-up), and ornamentation were a part of our ancestor's lives just as surely as they are today. Not so obviously, women chase men by arousing interest in specific males with social and sexual advances, what we call flirting. Women are skilled navigators of social scenarios. They do not flirt the same way with every man, but do so with great care and strategy. They avoid and repel men they are uninterested in; yet, at the same time, they attract and entice suitable mates, even outside of their primary partner, for many reasons: to inflate their self-worth, ignite jealousy in their lovers, increase attraction in their lovers, demonstrate their social capital, or to win a higher value mate. This fact, that women hunt, coupled with the biological reality of male libido, makes men easy prey for the advances of women, enabling women to go after specific males, which balances the romantic power of male agency, perhaps even exceeding it.

Attraction is the Response to Signals of Fertility and Genetic Value

Female suitability in regard to mate choice is based on several factors, but most notably, fertility. A fertile female is more likely to carry on the male's genetic heritage, and thus, feminine traits that signal fertility are the ones men evolved to prefer. These include waist-to-hip ratio, bust size, skin clarity, facial symmetry, bone structure, limb length, and more.

The formation of many of these physical indicators of fertility is due directly to a woman's health. Hormones levels throughout the developmental period, healthy stressors that aid development (such as exercise and macular activity), and even the social and emotional encounters that affect personality — all of these are examples of how environment comes to fulfill one's genetic potential. So, in a way, we are most attracted to those who are most well.

Why the difference in sex drive between men and women? Sex cells and the cost of reproduction. Men produce endless sperm cells while women lose most of their eggs by age 30. This fact predicts that men give theirs away more freely while women are more careful with theirs. Also, while the male's role in reproduction can take as little as a few minutes, the female's contribution can take years through pregnancy and child-rearing. Because of these biological differences and the increased cost of reproduction, women have evolved interesting tactics in regard to mate selection.

During peak fertility (ovulation), women tend to choose men who themselves display 'good genes', mostly as indicated by testosterone levels during puberty, a potent indicator of good health and survivability (procurement of food, immune system, ability to defend, etc.). However, when not at peak fertility, we see a phenomenon in female mate preference. That is, women prefer men who are slightly less 'manly' in the physical sense. Why would this be?

Women bear great cost of reproduction. Because of this, they have evolved a dual-plan of reproduction that increases the likelihood of choosing strong, resourceful mates that will bond and stay to care for the young, despite preferring more masculine men during peak fertility. They have elastic preferences, which increase the survival of her children and therefore the survival of her genes. The implication is a nefarious one, of course, because it describes the evolutionary advantage of tricking a male to raise another's children. On the other hand, maintaining bonds with a paternal figure vastly improves the survival fitness of her young, so there is a balance that must be found. Risking the loss of a paternal figure can have drastic consequences for her and her young.

Because women bear much of the responsibility of child-rearing, men have evolved a comparatively simple system of reproduction. Men display less choosiness over mates, instead responding via physical attraction to signs of fertility more broadly. There simply isn't a need for men to be selective in evolutionary terms, since women are selective for them, bearing most of the responsibility of child-rearing out of the necessity of pregnancy.

These competing systems between males and females increase the odds of survival for their children, but also increase the likelihood of eventual discord between the male-female pair, due to the competing desires of each person. This discord reveals why men and women cheat, albeit for different reasons. From an evolutionary perspective, taking a temporary, secondary partner grants a survival advantage for one's genetic material because an additional mate increases the odds of passing on genes. This has bestowed our modern selves with an admittedly dark element of human nature, and has led to very modern problems, like adultery, divorce, political scandals, and broken families. (Remember the 'naturalistic fallacy': natural, therefore good? Examples like cheating demonstrate exactly why it's a fallacy.)

But despite their competing interests in mating, reproduction, and child-rearing, men and women seek pair-bonds, which most biologists call monogamy. Perhaps this is not monogamy in the Disney sense of the word, but certainly in the biological sense of forming a primary pair-bond. (We will refine this concept in a coming section.) Monogamy-like behavior is observed among the vast majority of humans on the planet today. As we will see, society is structured just the right way to make this our default choice. But first, more on hormones.

Hormones of Romance

Lust is the immediate phase of romance. It is regulated primarily by the sex hormones, testosterone and estrogen. In men and women, testosterone triggers sex drive. Because testosterone levels are higher in men, they tend to play the role of pursuer. For this reason, modern culture depicts men as the gender responsible for making moves. However, estrogen plays an important role as well because it's what triggers attraction and the release of testosterone, all based on the estrogen levels of the female both of age and earlier during puberty, a critical time in her development. Estrogen is responsible for heightening her voice pitch in puberty and throughout each menstrual cycle,[299] developing her waist-to-hip ratio,[300] and growing her breasts. Together, these sex hormones create a climate ripe with lust for suitable

---

[299] Pipitone and Gallup (2008). Women's voice attractiveness varies across the menstrual cycle. *Evolution and Human Behavior* 29 (4): 268-274.

[300] Singh, Devendra (1993). Adaptive significance of female physical attractiveness: role of waist-to-hip ratio. *Journal of Personality and Social Psychology* 65 (2): 293-307.

mates.

Men prefer women that had high levels of estrogen during puberty, and women likewise tend to prefer men that had high levels of testosterone during puberty — which forges strong mating signals in men like facial hair, cranial shape, broad shoulders, and muscle mass. For women, selecting a mate isn't quite as simple as relying on physical indicators of health.

Women respond to cues beyond the physical. While women do consider the health of the male, they also place importance on social status and resources. This is due to the survival advantage of keeping a male during and after pregnancy that can protect, provide, and aid in child-rearing. By choosing a male with the qualities of a good father, females increase the odds that their genes will live on in their children. In this way, women are 'sexually selecting' for fatherly traits in males.

Resources, however, are not the only object of a woman's affection. His genes are. Evolution predicts that women are interested in genetic value. Thus, women are not attracted to men because they have resources, but rather, they are also attracted to men capable of winning resources. This draws a distinction between the arbitrary objects of the physical world and a man's genetic material, and it refines the old idea that women like men with money.

But that doesn't mean that women like 'alpha males', as so many popularly believe. In fact, alpha males are largely a myth. The image itself is one of dominance: the biggest, meanest, toughest. Like we see in wolfpacks. This may seem analogous, but humans are not wolves. In fact, anthropologists have illustrated precisely the opposite in natural social formations. As anthropologist Peter Gray says, "Anthropologists make it clear that hunter-gatherers were not passively egalitarian, but fiercely."[301] The theory describes a system of "reverse dominance," where even nuanced dominant behaviors are

---

[301] Gray, Peter (2010). How Hunter-Gatherers Maintained Their Egalitarian Ways: Three Complementary Theories. *Psychology Today* [Web file]Retrieved from http://www.psychologytoday.com/blog/freedom-learn/201105/how-hunter-gatherers-maintained-their-egalitarian-ways-three-complementary

squelched by the rest of the tribe members.[302] This is an idea that is applicable today, because people often don't enjoy the company of those who exhibit dominant behaviors. Many overbearing, forceful personalities achieve a false sense of status at the cost of the group's acceptance. Natural human social hierarchies are based on higher virtues than dominance and coercion.

Smell also plays a role in attraction. One of the best illustrations of the unseen influence of scent is how women in groups will begin ovulating at the same time when they spend long periods of time together. The evolutionary perspective to do so makes perfect sense, because it's a reproductive advantage to have all the males competing for all the women, rather than all the males competing for only a few women at a time.

Surprisingly, ovulation also plays a role in male and female arousal. Men tend to prefer women who are ovulating over those who are not. A UCLA study found that ovulating lap dancers made significantly more in tips than non-ovulating dancers, and dramatically more than menstruating dancers.[303] The authors of this study highlight that this may indicate human estrus, the male preference for women when they are most fertile. It may also, however, simply demonstrate how heightened female sexuality during ovulation may lead to greater male interest through flirting. Either way, the example fits an evolutionary perspective, because ovulating females are the ones most likely to succeed in reproduction.

Ovulation has also been shown to spur behavioral changes in men and women. Women who are closer to ovulation tend to dress more seductively than women who are not,[304] perhaps demonstrating a subconscious desire to fulfill their heightened reproductive potential. Women also fantasize more about non-primary partners when near ovulation, and men are more attentive to and protective of their partners during the peak fertility phase of

---

[302] Boehm, Christopher. *Hierarchy in the Forest: The Evolution of Egalitarian Behavior.* Harvard, 2001.

[303] Miller et al (2007). Ovulatory effects on tips earnings by lap dancers: economic evidence for human estrus? *Evolution and Human Behavior* 28 (6): 375-381.

[304] Haselton et al (2007). Ovulatory shifts in human female ornamentation: near ovulation, women dress to impress. *Hormones and Behavior* 51 (1): 41-45.

their partner's cycle.[305] Clearly, men are not consciously aware of their partner's cycles, so much of the song and dance of love takes place in the shadows of our minds.

Some scientists define attraction as the stage beyond simple lust, where the first deep connections and cravings are formed. These feelings are driven by dopamine, the hormone in the brain that plays a role in reward and motivation. In a popular 2005 study, people that were "in love" were observed to have heightened activity in the reward and motivation segments of the brain when viewing photographs of their loved ones.[306] These results were confirmed in studies of separate populations.[307] This points to evolved bio-mechanisms that drive people to focus their attention towards individual mates during the intense early stage of love. This initial romantic stage is critical for mate selection, in particular, the survival of offspring.

The dopamine bio-mechanism is so potent that it remains activated even if the individual is rejected by their lover. In a 2010 study by Helen Fisher at Rutgers University, people who were recently rejected yet still "in love" were observed to have activated mesolimbic reward/survival systems, suggesting that romantic passion exists for those who are happily and unhappily in love.[308] The activation of systems implicated in cocaine addiction may explain the deep feelings of attachment that persist through time and the obsessive behavior commonly seen with the rejection of love.

Sex and love take place in different areas of the brain. While sexual desire is activated in the same place as food and drugs, the area activated by love is the part of the brain involved in conditioning behavior based on reward or

---

[305] Gangestad, Thornhill, and Garver (2002). Changes in women's sexual interests and their partners mate-retention tactics across the menstrual cycle. *Proceedings of the Royal Society Biological Sciences* 269 (1494): 975-982.

[306] Aron et al (2005). Reward, Motivation, and Emotion Systems associated with early stage intense romantic love. *Journal of Neurophysiology* 94 (1): 327-337.

[307] Xu et al (2011). Reward and motivation systems: a brain mapping study of early stage romantic love in Chinese participants. *Human Brain Mapping* 32 (2): 237-249.

[308] Fisher et al (2011). Reward, addiction, and emotion regulation systems associated with rejection in love. *Journal of Neurophysiology* 104 (1): 51-60.

pleasure.[309] Things that trigger reward or pleasure over time are given inherent value, just like an addiction. As psychologist Jim Pfaus explains, "Love is actually a habit that is formed from sexual desire as desire is rewarded. It works the same way in the brain as when people become addicted to drugs."[310] A broken heart can be seen as a withdrawal from a strong addiction. In light of this evidence, it's easy to see how the brain can drive obsession. Obsession has been observed to detract from the satisfaction of the relationship and the length of the relationship.[311] Together, these might hold clues on why heartbreak is one of the most painful human experiences, and perhaps what to do about it.

Many partners stay together after early-stage romantic love. In fact, long-term relationships have long been known to be based on deep bonds rooted in companionship, friendship, and memory. However, science confirms that romantic love persists in the long term, fueling feelings of love well beyond that of mere companionship and friendship.[312] These findings speak volumes about the unique nature of human bonding and mating strategies in an evolutionary context. If human beings evolved to form persisting romantic feelings for long-term partners, then the implications are huge for many aspects of modern life. Evolutionary theory predicts that a bio-mechanism must exist that would promote long-term feelings of love.

Well, we've found one in vasopressin, which is implicated in the long-term bonds formed by lovers.[313] Vasopressin is a hormone, some of which is excreted by the brain, where it plays an important role in pair bonding and

[309] Cacioppo et al (2012). The common neural bases between sexual desire and love: a multilevel kernel density fMRI analysis. *The Journal of Sexual Medicine* 9 (4): 1048.

[310] ScienceDaily (2012). "I want to know where love is: first brain map of love and desire." [Web file] Retrieved from http://www.sciencedaily.com/releases/2012/06/120620101011.htm.

[311] Graham, James (2011). Measuring love in romantic relationships: a meta-analysis. *Journal of Social and Personal Relationships* 28 (6): 748-771.

[312] Acevedo and Aron (2009). Does a long-term relationship kill romantic love? *Review of General Psychology* 13 (1): 59.

[313] Carter and Porges (2010). Social bonding and attachment. *Encyclopedia of Behavioral Neuroscience.*

male paternal care. Much of what we know about the hormone is thanks to a rodent called the prairie vole. Like humans, voles engage in long-term monogamy, which is fairly rare in nature. When scientists disturb the vasopressin brain system, they find that voles end their monogamous ways and neglect their child-rearing duties.[314] Vasopressin also may play a role in mate guarding, because it's been shown to drive aggression.[315] Together these things are clear indicators of the biological basis for long-term mating, perhaps indicating that humans are built to handle long-term partners.

Love is Real

> Gravitation cannot be held responsible for people falling in love. How on earth can you explain in terms of chemistry and physics so important a biological phenomenon as first love? Put your hand on a stove for a minute and it seems like an hour. Sit with that special girl for an hour and it seems like a minute. That's relativity.
>
> **Albert Einstein**, god of nerds

It boggles my mind that there are people in the world that don't believe in love. Evolution requires coming to terms with many dark truths about human nature. It explains why people cheat, murder, lie, steal, and deceive. But this is one area where a disconnected society's cynicism has run riot on some people's ability to bond with others, detracting from their quality of life.

Just listen to popular music or watch an old western film and you'll inevitably come across a male flaunting his ability to keep women at an emotional distance. For young men coming of age, these ideas may become

---

[314] Wang et al (1998). Voles and vasopressin: a review of cellular, molecular, and behavioral studies of pair bonding and paternal behavior. *Progress in Brain Research* 119: 483-499.

[315] Young, Wang, and Inzel (1998). Neuroendocrine bases for monogamy. *Trends in Neurosciences* 21 (2): 71-5.

part of their perspective on the world. There are many men who accept, as part of their masculinity, the disconnect from what they want and what they feel. This is the lie some people live every day.

And how are women supposed to react? Predictably, they put up defenses against threatening, selfish acts by men. Without trust, sexual access is further complicated. Every man is looked upon with suspicion and kept at a distance, only furthering the cultural mythology of gender. The strong hand of culture divides men and women beyond the biological, because many people forget that love is real, that men and women really just want the same things, with subtle differences.

Love is essentially an extension of the human reproductive system. It is as real as it gets.

The hormonal regulation of behaviors surrounding love highlights the complexity behind love as an evolved trait. It paints a picture of a strongly emotional species, one capable of boundless love and affection. As anthropologist Helen Fisher says, "We are programmed to love multiple people at the same time." This is indeed the truth of love that is explored in poetry, film, books, and art, but not commonly accepted to have an evolutionary basis.

It's this boundless love that gets us into trouble. Often, men and women who cheat are publicly shamed, labeled as abnormal, misguided, or even evil. So how, then, do many couples manage to get through stable marriages faithfully? Is their resistance to natural urges stronger? Or are their impulses to stay together likewise driven by evolution? As we shall see in the next chapter, the foundations for human morality may be rooted more deeply than many folks realize, undoubtedly implicated in the virtue of long-term companionship. And while our very nature can sometimes be at odds with our well-being, there are some curiously natural inclinations that drive us to be noble, virtuous, and just plain good.

But first, let's call into question the assumption that human beings are naturally monogamous, which in strict terms becomes dubious in the face of the evidence.

The Standard Narrative of Evolutionary Sciences

When it comes to classifying human behavior, scientists reach an almost insurmountable challenge due to the complex multitude of behaviors, norms, and values across many different human societies. How do we define what is natural in complex realms, and harder still, how do we define what is natural in controversial realms? Sexuality is perhaps the most challenging subject of all due to its social stigma, cultural politics, and biological complexity.

So where are we now? Most evolutionary sciences have, almost prematurely, nailed down the answer to human sexuality. They have defined us as serial monogamists who seek out extra-pair copulation when it suits us, men looking to scatter their seed and women looking to procure a more valuable sperm donor. In this model, nuclear families are important, fidelity is respected, and the status quo is upheld. Sound familiar? It should. This model of human sexuality is the Disney version of love, mixed with the tumult of modern relationships, the crumbling nuclear families, and garnished with the patriarchal values of the puritans of old.

Serial monogamists, but we have sex with other people, too. See how the very definition already points away from monogamy? Why would we have simultaneous needs to form a long term partner and take on additional partners? Why are we even capable of loving multiple people at once?

To its credit, this model of sexuality is close to the mark in evolutionary biology, where the puzzle of human sexual behavior is difficult to solve. Indeed many of the puzzle pieces fit. Evolutionary biology, after all, is precisely the place to look for answers to these questions. The problem is that biology alone does not fully encapsulate human behavior. To understand evolution is to add another vitally important ingredient to the recipe of human behavior that clears up the fog in the standard narrative, because we can see clearly in the light of evolution that humans have social architecture built atop biological architecture, and this fact changes the flavor of our favorite dish.

The Sexual Lives of Social Beings

"The social lives of foragers are characterized by a depth and intensity of interaction few of us could imagine (or tolerate). For those of us born and raised in societies organized around the interlocking principles of individuality, personal space, and private property, it's difficult to project our imaginations into those tightly woven societies where almost all space and property is communal, and identity is more collective than individual. From the first morning of birth to the final mourning of death, a forager's life is one of intense, constant interaction, interrelation, and interdependence."

Christopher Ryan and Cacilda Jethá, shame exorcists

I'll say it: human beings are the most highly evolved social organism in the history of life on Earth. We have the most complex social networks, the richest palette of emotion, and are the first species to coagulate into groups of groups. While other social animals rival our numbers and our reproductive success, our social nature is what enabled our survival in the wild and what propels us to the heights of progress today.

Marrying our social nature to our sexual prowess, and understanding how human nature, forged in the ancestral environment, was adopted and indoctrinated by civilization, helps us to understand sexual behavior today, and sexual behavior as it evolved. It is the social architecture built atop our biological architecture that illuminates the mysteries and complexities of human sexuality.

Environment Changes Everything

Environment matters greatly to the behavior of an organism. Say you have a group of chimpanzees, and you give them a ton of bananas; these chimps will share in the environment of abundance and remain relatively peaceful and egalitarian. Now say that you throw them a single banana; they will fight over it, form dominance hierarchies, and behave relatively malevolently in the face of scarcity. Simply shifting the environment from abundance to scarcity greatly affects their behavior. In a similar way, civilization has done so with human sexuality.

Feminism is perhaps the most potent academic discipline to have unraveled the systems of power in civilization that dominate, oppress, suppress, and repress its citizens, both men and women. As such, it is a valuable perspective on how systems of power vie with human nature. When married with evolution, the interpretations are potent. Regarding sexuality, it illuminates the ways civilization retards our sexual development, quelches our sexual expression, shames our sexual needs, and pathologizes our sexual nature.

Take a simple look at what we do, even in the "advanced" Western world. We show pictures of rotting genitals to our children to instill fear in their hearts about sex, and we call it sex education. We mutilate genitals at birth to curb masturbation when boys come of age, and we call it circumcision. We tell our girls that if they like sex they're sluts, and our boys that if they have feelings they're queer. Girls are raised to be coy and asexual, closed to every suitor, and openly encouraged to use their sexuality coercively. Culture teaches our boys to spread their seed unscrupulously, without attachment or concern for the feelings of others. We romanticize love in Disney movies and anesthetize love in rap music. Popular culture teaches arbitrary gender roles that echo a dark oppressive history of puritanical sexuality, class warfare, and false gender identity.

We create a romantic scenario based on competition rather than cooperation, secrecy rather than openness, ownership rather than sharing, politics rather than pleasure, and coercion rather than mutual fulfillment. And then we wonder why people are lonely, couples bored, and hearts scarred. Do I really have to explain why this is unnatural? That this is not the environment that matches our evolution? That this has no bearing in science or reason? That even by historical standards this is shameful and oppressive and downright embarrassing? Alexis de Tocqueville once said, "It is easier to accept a simple lie than a complex truth." This is no different.

Our entire system of sex and love was inherited from puritanical forbears. It is their obsolete values rooted in patriarchy and fanaticism that echo in our culture today and touch us still. Their values, foreign to human nature, are so ubiquitous that many folks don't realize the degree to which we have already been indoctrinated. We simply accept our inheritance as an unquestionable cultural ethos, even despite the obvious truth that the Disney version of love doesn't always work. By the numbers, it mostly fails.

The standard system of sex and love falls flat on its face precisely *because* it is unnatural. Half of marriages don't last and many of those that do wallow in the doldrums of despondency. Even happy marriages leave people empty; somewhere around half of cheating spouses report that their marriages are "happy" or "very happy."[316] Everything that marriage is supposed to stand for (stability, security, commitment, tradition, duty, eternity, even passion) soon faces the crushing reality that we are animals and animals don't like cages. Our cultural ethos relies on the mythology of love, the dogma of nuclear family, and the subjugation of sex in order to persist. This model of society is outdated and only evolution explains why.

In the ancestral environment, human relationships were fluid, dynamic, and complex. They were defined by emotion, instinct, survival, group cohesion, status, fertility, compatibility, sharing, lust, love, obligation, morality, family, tribe, honor, and responsibility. For humans in the wild, social networks are expansive, a breadth and depth of connection that most are not even capable of comprehending, because the comforts of civilization, while valuable, also silently soften the depth of human bonds.

Imagine what the bonds are like among gangsters, pitted against the world, reliant on their homeboys for their very lives, or among soldiers,

---

[316] Glass and Wright (1985). Sex differences in type of extramarital involvement and marital dissatisfaction. *Sex Roles* 12 (9-10): 1101-1120.

fighting for each other at the doorsteps of hell, or even among dance troupes, united by a daunting performance and years of physical intimacy, and maybe you'll get close to understanding the depths of a true human bond and how that bond comes to define human sexuality. Adversity is unifying. In society, where is our group identity? Our adversity?

Group Identity is Dead For Most People and,

With It, a Network of Lovers

The truth is that sex is a bonding mechanism. In the words of Christopher Ryan and Cacilda Jethá, sex "strengthens the bonds among individuals in small-scale nomadic societies (and, apparently, other highly interdependent groups), forming a crucial, durable web of affection, affiliation, and mutual obligation."[317] In their landmark pop science book, *Sex at Dawn*, Ryan and Jethá present a crucial new hypothesis to explain human sexuality: the sex act is about bonding, not simply reproduction. And the more you look at sexual behavior, even deviant forms, the more this seems to be true. The more questions posed, the more obvious this fact becomes.

Why do people in grief seek out sex? Why do over a third of people cheat? Why are up to a third of children fathered illegitimately?[318] Why does so much pornography feature group sex? Why are our most vexing fantasies and temptations with people we know, rather than strangers who are more genetically fit? Why do women beg for sexual attention from men they would never sleep with? Why are women (and men[319]) capable of multiple orgasms? Why is watching others have sex so arousing? Why is estrus, a woman's fertile period, comparatively hidden in humans? Why is rape more likely committed by someone we know, and more perplexingly, even by someone we love? Why do we copulate year-round? Why do other primates and

---

[317] Ryan and Jethá, pp 93-94.

[318] Meller, William. *Evolution Rx*. Penguin, 2009. p 182.

[319] Dunn and Trost (1989). Male multiple orgasms: a descriptive study. *Archives of Sexual Behavior* 18: 377-387.

mammals last seconds without thrusting while humans last several minutes, even hours, with it? Why do women moan loudly during sex? Why do their ovulatory cycles inevitably coincide? None of the answers to these questions can be fully understood unless you look at them in the light of evolution; the picture of a group-living primate having sex in the context of bonding adequately, and almost easily, explains these mysteries. As the legendary biologist E.O. Wilson once said, "All that we can surmise of humankind's genetic history argues for a more liberal sexual morality, in which sexual practices are to be regarded first as bonding devices and only second as a means of procreation."[320]

Three Chimps and a Mysterious Ancestor

The closest relatives to humans are chimpanzees and bonobos (often called pygmy chimps). Our DNA differs only by 1.6 percent from each of them. Interestingly, both are highly promiscuous. At peak, they have sex multiple times per day with several different lovers. Albeit, they do so in very different ways.

Bonobos are egalitarian and peaceful, maintaining ties primarily through social bonding by females and secondarily through social bonding between females and males. Bonds are long-term, allowing a cooperative and intensive mating network typified by sex. Lots of sex of all kinds. Bonobos engage in sex so regularly that they use it to diffuse tension, obtain pleasure, and bond. Females often rub their genitals together as a normal part of socializing. They are the only other animal from humans to stare longingly into each other's eyes and kiss deeply.[321]

Chimps are a fascinating counter-example, because their promiscuity is achieved instead through dominance, coercion, and hierarchy. Chimps form constantly shifting male coalitions that patrol the females in their territory.

---

[320] Wilson, EO. *On Human Nature.* Harvard, 2012. p 142.
[321] Ryan and Jethá, pp 77-78.

Females do not form bonds with other females or any particular male.[322] Disturbingly, the chimpanzee model has been favored in the interpretation of natural human sexual behavior. But is it fair to call humans chimps?

Humans, the third chimp relative that descended from the common ancestor five million years ago, in addition to the bonobo, exhibits many behaviors that encapsulate both the bonobo and the chimp. Both males and females bond strongly with their own sex, but females are slightly more intelligent socially. Some believe this may point to matriarchy in humans, creating an environment where "males tend to fare pretty well," much like bonobo males do.[323] Moreover, female sexuality is malleable, shaped by the culture and environment that contains it. Women have been shown to become aroused by a wide range of stimuli, a testament to the diversity and potency of human sexuality, and one that points away from the standard model of monogamy.[324]

The common ancestor between humans, chimps, and bonobos has yet to be discovered, but picturing an ape that shares the characteristics of all the animals above should say something, should it not? Promiscuity is seen in all of these species, so the common ancestor must have laid the groundwork for this behavior. It was ultimately the environment of civilization that makes it hard to decode human sexuality and to gauge what is natural.

"Just imagine that we had never heard of chimpanzees or baboons and had known bonobos first. We would at present most likely believe that early hominids lived in female-centered societies, in which sex served important social functions and in which warfare was rare or absent."

Frans de Waal, bonobo researcher

---

[322] Ryan and Jethá, pp 66-67.

[323] Ryan and Jethá, p 71.

[324] Bergner, Daniel. *What Do Women Want? Adventures in the Science of Female Desire.* HarperCollins, 2013.

Swinging and Sharing: Environments Define Openness

Consider the well-known homoeroticism of the soldier. These young men and women, brought together against a common threat, forge deep bonds in battle. Their level of comfort with each other exceeds more than most people will ever understand or experience in a group setting. What's interesting is how their sexuality surfaces in their behavior, how they flirt with each other in socially appropriate ways, reference sex often, are comfortable with nudity, precisely because they are falling back on their sexuality as a bonding mechanism, even against the grave taboo of homosexuality that culture teaches. It is well known in military circles that soldiers go into battle as much for each other as anything else, because they become tribe, an emotional proximity that many people subject to the comforts of society will never know or understand. Not convinced?

Swinging almost certainly started on military bases. Pilots during World War II would throw parties before deployment, and this is where the first known partner swapping occurred. It was understood that some men would not return from war, and there was a tacit gentlemen's understanding that those men's families would be taken care of. Sex was the mechanism that drove and reflected those bonds, creating the apt environment for support and care. Does evolution explain why soldiers at war would more easily open and share their sexuality than others? Perhaps it does.

In the wild, dangers lurk at every corner. Until about 10,000 years ago, there were saber-toothed cats circling the perimeters of human encampments. Dire wolves and American lions hunted the same lands as humans, as did short-faced bears, the fastest bear of all time, weighing in at 1500 pounds. There was the mystery of disease, high infant mortality, life-threatening injuries, and the threat of strangers and neighboring clans — all of which likely brought the tribe members closer to the reality of death, to an understanding of life's daily peril, and to an emotional proximity to one another. They relied on each other in ways most can't even comprehend.

Almost no one in modern society knows what it's like to have to belong to a group, to belong or die. Almost no one knows what it's like to exist in a place where death haunts you, often reminding you of its proximity by killing babies, eating people alive, or casting the mysterious spell of disease. Almost no one knows how the adversity of the wild drives people into the arms and hearts of others as a simple matter of survival. The "grizzly man" Timothy Treadwell lived among bears for years before he was eaten alive. This is a wild death, a death by natural causes. Grief drives us into the arms of others because it reminds us that death isn't just coming, it's already here. The soft minds of society struggle to forget this fact. It doesn't fit their worldview of charming princes, angels, and yoga pants.

In the wild, you are always days away from death. You'll last three days without water, two weeks without food. If sick or injured, you'll need help from a number of people. This environment shaped group identity and necessitated loyalty, cooperation, mastery, sharing, egalitarianism, and love. Imagine having a dozen people who would kill or die for you at the drop of a hat, men who protected your loved ones, women who cared for you, all of whom shared everything and meant everything. Do you really think that in this group only one person at a time would excite you sexually? Would you mind sharing if everyone was already sharing with you?

Human egalitarianism is rooted in sharing. Our ancestors took sharing to be a fundamental matter of principle, a core construct of morality. As Matt Ridley writes,

> ...all human beings share a fascinating taboo...the taboo against selfishness. Selfishness is almost the definition of vice. Murder, theft, rape, and fraud are considered crimes of great importance because they are selfish or spiteful acts that are committed for the benefit of the actor and the detriment of the victim. In contrast, virtue is, almost by definition, the greater good of the group.[325]

---

[325] Ridley, Matt. *The Origins of Virtue.* p 38.

Human ancestors in the wild took for granted freedom, egalitarianism, and personal autonomy because they *were* granted. Mother Nature grants these in their entirety. Only other people are capable of taking them away. Does it stand to reason that sex, too, is shared?

The environment that frames the portrait of human sexuality could not be more different than the environment of civilization. Some populations today, like soldiers, mirror some elements of the ancestral environment. In the case of the soldier, facing death and a common enemy, omnipresent in the ancestral environment, nurtured the bonds between them and changed the game of human sexuality, making them more likely to share partners, whether that be openly, tacitly, ritualistically, or secretly, to create larger networks of love, and to have their needs, sexual and emotional, fully met.

Compare this to today's world of mating. In a city full of strangers, you get one partner at a time if you're lucky, all while probably lacking close, lifelong friendships and being displaced from your family and childhood friends due to the demands of school, career, or life. Many acquaintances are, by necessity, kept at an emotional distance, never truly knowing the person underneath the career persona. Today's environment makes monogamy viable precisely because it reduces the options and incentivizes forming a single pair bond instead of a primary pair bond.

Rather than having only one lover, our ancestors more likely participated in a shifting, interconnected hierarchy of lovers, much like we do with friends, which included multiple pair bonds. Women literally evolved to attract potential mates at all times from every direction; each additional suitor, even without sex, is a boon to her survival and, with sex, to her survival *and* reproductive fitness. Attraction is a woman's insurance plan, mate-guarding strategy, and status symbol all at once. This is the only thing that makes sense of a woman's obsession with attracting sexual attention via beauty and flirtation. Even after marriage, women are still highly sexualized, exerting great effort to remain beautiful (as any plastic surgeon can attest), gladly walking the lines of socially appropriate flirtation, and taking extra lovers nearly as often as men (sometimes more[326]), whether that be openly, tacitly, ritualistically, or secretly.

Any investor can explain why putting all your eggs in one basket is a bad idea, which is exactly what happens with modern love. Any zoologist can tell you how scarcity spurs negative behaviors in primates, which is exactly what happens with modern love. Where there should be a vast network of family, friends, and lovers, for many there is only a deified One. For some, everything is invested into one partner, and when that stock falls, the ensuing loss is more than any person should experience, more than any natural relationship should endure. It's more than some can bear, and its mental, social, and emotional consequences eternal.

What is Love? (The Remix)

Framed in the light of this new social bonding hypothesis, what then does love become? How can we define true love if it's not simply the religious Disney version that we are spoon-fed as children? There is a simple answer: love is the bond between people. And there is a more nuanced answer: love is the glue of group cohesion.

There are only two good reasons why humans are good at life. Clearly, we are. We pretty much conquered the planet so well that it's become a problem. But why? And how? We're not fast, not very strong. We don't have sharp claws and teeth. So what gives?

All of the power of our species stems from the fact that we are smart and social. Our intellect and sociality contribute greatly to our ability to adapt and unify. These are the twin pillars under which we have constructed the greatest apparatus of life in the known universe: civilization. And they are leading us into a mysterious and imposing future.

Love enables group cohesion by creating a dynamic, interconnected

---

[326] Brand et al (2007). Sex differences in self-reported infidelity and its correlates. *Sex Roles* 57(1-2):101-109.

network of individuals. The more bonds, and the stronger those bonds, the stronger the group. Thus, evolution predicts that social animals must have mechanisms that drive group bonding. As arguably the most elevated social animals, humans have many.

Categories of human bonding include talking, touching, sharing, cooperating, giving, playing, experiencing, and copulating. Of these, sex is the most potent. It is capable of strengthening a bond to psychotropic levels, the heights of which are only truly captured by art and poetry. We look each other in the eye when we talk, and we look each other in the eye when we make love. No other animal does both of these things, and the only one that does it while mating is the bonobo, our closest relative, who is well known as a group-living, promiscuous species that uses sex to maintain a network of relationships.

Natural Human Bonding Strategies

Talking	Telling stories, sharing feelings, trusting secrets, learning about others, giving compliments, achieving familiarity
Touching	Greeting (hugging, kissing, shaking hands), grooming, cuddling, massaging, holding hands, comforting
Sharing	Food, water, resources, ideas, relationships (connections, friends, lovers)
Cooperating	Helping others in a common goal, leading and supporting others' lead, protecting
Giving	Gifts, favors, experiences
Playing	Joking around, playing games, being silly, dancing, roughhousing, practical jokes, pranks
Experiencing	Art, music, ritual, travel, recreational substances, danger, grief, solidarity, pleasure
Copulating	Do I really need to give examples here?

Consider casual sex, which many people label as unemotional. How casual and unemotional is it really? A third of casual encounters on dating sites end up in long-term relationships.[327] Think about that. That means that out of a whole bunch of sexually and socially repressed people, who are so desperate for sex that they will turn to strangers on the internet, up to a third will find love despite the fact that they have openly agreed to something casual, the opposite of what would be romantic, emotional, and fulfilling.

---

[327] Helen Fisher mentioned this statistic from the Match.com Singles in America Study on her microblog with the comment, "Casual sex: not so casual!"

And what about the sex that is *actually* casual? Certainly, some people are built to seek and prefer casual sex, and many do it in a way that is safe and healthy. But this usually occurs between people who are already acquainted. And if they are not, there is always a period, however brief, of building rapport and achieving familiarity and trust, whether that be a few dances, a date, an introduction, or a good conversation. Even prostitutes banter before the transaction, and many see return customers who stay in touch. It may be casual, but it's certainly not a sex act devoid of human sociality.

Speaking of transactions: love can add an important part to the formula of romance. If you recall the old idea that women trade sexual access for a man's resources, then you might be reminded of the prostitute in the previous paragraph. Are we meant to think of all women as whores? Fortunately not, because this shadowy concept is seen more clearly in the light of the social bonding hypothesis. Now, the transaction needs a middleman; emotion becomes the currency in the economics of love. A woman has sex with a man because she loves him. A man provides resources for a woman because he loves her. And vice versa, obviously. A man has sex with a woman because he loves her. A woman provides for a man because she loves him.

Sex ↔ Love ↔ Resources

The good news is that this perfectly fits contemporary ideals of appropriate sexual behavior. In our culture today, a man is okay to have sex in pretty much any scenario. But if a woman has sex with a man for money, she's a whore. If she has sex for fun, she's a slut. It's only for love that a woman is not shamed or stigmatized. So this happens to jive quite well with our conception of what is healthy, proper sexual behavior. Sex in the context of bonding — a lucky beam in the light and shadows of evolutionary interpretation.

So if humans are not naturally monogamous, then what are they? The answer is that humans are naturally polyamorous, built to feel many kinds of love for many kinds of people, and any number of those people are going to have sexual chemistry with each other in the right context. We have different kinds of love for our pets, parents, children, friends, mentors, and lovers. It is one love that bonds us together, but it is a multi-faceted love that manifests itself uniquely to each relationship. Sexuality is awakened when the context is right, when a suitable mate is identified. This may be one, could be none, but it's more likely to be a number of special relationships, each one challenging and chaotic, yet at the same time meaningful, fulfilling, and profound. The hard question is what to do about it.

We all grew up in a specific era of a civilized society where most group identity is dead. We did not grow up in the wild. Our decision about what to do with this new understanding of sexuality is especially puzzling and complex. It may be that practicing polyamory in the environment of civilization is a bit like practicing monogamy in the wild; the behavior must fit the environment. For many of us, it's too late, too radical. We have already accepted the burden of shame that society passes down. But at the same time we live in a society full of endless possibilities and many different types of people, cultures, and value systems. Does that make polyamory possible?

The truth is that most people do what is comfortable and easy. Most will probably stick with the traditional system; luckily, it works for many. It's the most incentivized option, financially and otherwise. Given the environment of today's society, it's the simplest and easiest because it's the standard. On the other hand, some are more comfortable risking an unconventional lifestyle. They will find their own middle ground. Perhaps they date around, or perhaps they cheat. Perhaps they open their relationship, or perhaps they experiment while they're young. Perhaps they practice serial monogamy, perhaps they are better off alone. Embracing diversity is the new theme of a contemporary understanding of human sexuality.

Evolution predicts that the most important traits develop the most complexity and variation. Since reproduction is the cornerstone of evolution, sexuality is probably the most complex and varied part of the human genome. This is why each person's sexuality is its own labyrinth to explore, unique as a fingerprint, and each person's goals will flow where the many forces in life guide it. With hope, coming to know the truth about one's own sexuality is a force for positive change. And, at the very least, it's damn interesting.

Jealousy is fuel for managing relationships. Let it burn.

Any manager worth their salt will tell you that fear is the best motivator, but what they may not know is how and why biological channels for fear evolved in humans. A lot of fear is easy to understand, such as in the fight-or-flight response, but the most interesting kind of fear is jealousy, because it serves as motivational fuel for managing human relationships.

Consider friendship. Networks of friends are ever-changing, waxing and waning according to the chaos and bustle of life. Your best friend today may not be your best friend in five years and may not be your best friend five years ago. Your best friend may have a best friend who is not you. They may have two or three best friends, including or excluding you. Almost everyone has lost a friend or seen a friendship diminish. Almost everyone knows what it must feel like to lose their place among friends, to be left out of a group outing, or to share a friend they want all to themselves. That feeling fuels action. In friendships, jealousy can motivate finding more friends, deepening bonds with current friends, or winning respect among high-status members of the group. As such, jealousy, along with many other emotions, plays a crucial role in managing all kinds of relationships.

The role that jealousy plays is in motivating individuals to re-establish, compete for, and grow the bonds that are important to them, and it's an emotion that includes all or most of the social network, not merely lovers. So in this way, we are constantly managing feelings about, say, strangers and acceptance, colleagues and promotions, parents and siblings, friends and status, lovers and sex. We want new people to accept us, our bosses to respect us, our friends to like us, our parents to be proud of us, and our lovers to love us. Jealousy helps us achieve those ends. Therefore, jealousy is not proof of monogamy, but rather one more interesting turn in the maze of human sexuality, and it's analogous to all relationships.

With lovers today, jealousy is artificially elevated because of the environment in which it operates: the scarce environment of monogamy that yields repression, pathology, shame, loneliness, and stigma. Societal conventions dictate that, in a world of strangers, we must accept only one lover; therefore, only one close friendship. As a consequence, culture enforces that fiction. It becomes inappropriate to pursue male-female friendships. We are wary of advances from strangers, suspicious of their motives. There is stigma to flirting too much, or doing something too intimate, or spending too much time, all lines that are arbitrarily drawn in the shifting sands of time. Thus, we are left with all eggs in one basket, a basket that breaks more often than not. We place importance on how long we have this basket, rather than how deep it goes. Predictably, we are inordinately protective of this basket, incentivized to keep others away from it and hoard it only for ourselves.

It is a sick twist of civilization to make normal owning other people. There are 20 million slaves in the world today, yet every single soul in society is owned in some way, whether by a bank, a corporation, or an unsuspecting spouse. Humans are born free and autonomous as a birthright, yet the Bible reads, "You shall not covet your neighbor's house. You shall not covet your neighbor's wife, or his manservant or maidservant, his ox or donkey, or anything that belongs to your neighbor." This sacred book is the root of modern marriage and it goads you to treat your best friend like property. Ryan and Jethá, who I have so thoroughly referenced, once again hit the mark:

> Some behaviors that seem normal to contemporary people (and which are therefore readily assumed to be universal) would quickly destroy many small-scale foraging societies, rendering them dysfunctional. Unrestrained self-interest, in particular, whether expressed as food-hoarding or excessive sexual possessiveness, is a direct threat to group cohesion and is therefore considered shameful and ridiculous.[328]

---

[328] Ryan and Jethá, p 139.

Should it come as a shock that humans are not meant to be possessed? That it is unnatural to consider another person to be yours? Why has our culture so readily accepted this norm? Why does it not fill us with the proportionate disgust of slavery or indentured servitude? Are we to accept the fact that the price of jealousy is one's freedom and independence?

Jealousy is not a problem, and even if it was, monogamy wouldn't solve it. Those who are in committed relationships still experience jealousy. There is no amount of promising, no type of ritual, including marriage, and no amount of legal paperwork that will totally ensure the security of a relationship. We all know that the basket breaks half the time. People change. People die. People steal, cheat, and lie. This is simply human nature and the nature of love. Looking to marriage as something that solves the jealousy problem is more an insight into the modern state of human connection, desperate and pathetic, than it is a form of emotional insurance.

Contemporary society and culture is structured and delivered in a way that takes jealousy to unnatural places, precisely because it is an unnatural system. It should be no wonder why an anthill full of lonely, tribeless, socially inept, and sexually repressed people, recent descendants of religious fanatics, heirs to a misogynistic patriarchy, would place so much importance on the sexual exclusivity of one partner. The more you need that partner, the more you need to need that partner. That's what monogamous marriage does. It provides the basket for all those eggs. The loneliest people need it most, yet it makes them lonelier. At the same time, the loneliest people tend to be the most jealous. Sadly, the most jealous people are making themselves lonelier in an unfortunate circle of pathology.

For those who think jealousy proves something about the validity of monogamy, what would its opposite prove? Because there is another human emotion called compersion, the empathetic state of positive feelings one experiences when someone they love experiences happiness, joy, or pleasure. Most often, it is a word used among polyamorists who find joy or pleasure in sharing their partners with others. You may have caught it in Woody Allen's film exploring the needs of love, *Vicky, Cristina, Barcelona*, or in the hit TV show *House of Cards*, starring Kevin Spacey and Robin Wright. How could this emotion exist alongside jealousy if our species was truly monogamous? Only evolution makes sense of how these two competing and compromising emotions coexist, shedding light on a natural human sexuality.

Civilization Makes Men and Women Enemies

The history of civilizational patriarchy explains why systems of power taught women to be chaste. As sex objects, virgins are more valuable. Consequently, culture enforces this value. Many women, even today, participate in slut-shaming. Every woman today dreams of her white wedding and some never suspect its nefarious origins (to become a man's property). Even those keen to feminism adapt its meaning, making it fit their worldview, perhaps compromising the ritual to make it work. Almost no one is able to reject a cultural institution so highly prized. Who can blame them? Culture is a powerful force, and the modern wedding has become sacred.

Predictably, this unnatural attitude toward women led men in the opposite direction. Thinking of women as possessions led men to objectify and dehumanize them. Many men considered women vessels for children and sex. Others thought of women as enemies to male need. The rift between men and women only further plundered their cooperation, leaving many today unfulfilled sexually and emotionally. Many boys today don't know how to talk to girls because this rift is so wide. Is it any wonder that men today still uphold the cultural value of unattached promiscuity? Is this not a perfect reaction to a woman's chastity? Two unnatural systems. Are we to believe that men evolved to spread their seed unscrupulously and women to close their heart to all but the best suitor? Clearly, a natural system for men and women would land somewhere in the middle.

This leaves us with three interesting scenarios among the many worth considering. Many people reading this may still be shocked at the idea that our species is highly sexual and emotional, so for them I present the following table. What our culture teaches some women and what our culture teaches some men are polarized. In the middle is polyamorous tribalism, what many today argue is the natural human sexuality. It highlights that civilization is what divides male and female needs. Under a natural system, men and women are both fulfilled. In a natural system, they both need the same things.

Traditional Monogamy (What ~~sheep~~ women want?)	Group Polyamory (What's ~~human~~ natural)	Independent Promiscuity (What ~~wolves~~ men want?)
Life-long commitment to a single partner	Fluid sexual and emotional attachment to any number of in-group partners	Unlimited sexual liaisons without attachment, commitment, or group relation
Nuclear family group unit serves as basic level of security. Simplicity may bolster stability. Mother and father rear children, many single parent households, some orphans. Rampant cheating amidst low rates of sexual fulfillment. Most incentivized option.	Strong group identity with sense of obligation to and affiliation with group members. Multiple parental figures and role models contribute to child-rearing. Cheating rates unclear, sexual and emotional fulfillment high. Perhaps disabled by modern environment.	Little to no group belonging. Little to no emotional proximity to others. Child-rearing of no concern. Cheating impossible since commitment never formed. Sexually satisfying, emotionally unfulfilling.

The cartoonist Hugh MacLeod once said, "The price of being a sheep is boredom. The price of being a wolf is loneliness. Choose one or the other with great care." But what about the third option? What is the price of being human, where lonliness and boredom are cured? Why have we not even considered a system that matches our social evolution? Today's culture is so far removed from nature that being human isn't even considered an option, because our popular consciousness does not understand what it means to be human, and the environment in which we live disables that option. Perhaps time and knowledge will change that.

Strategies in Sex and Love

Attraction is simply the response to signals of fertility and genetic value. It's not just about the body, but also the brain. A clever quip, a good deed, a funny joke, balanced energy, graceful communication or mannerisms, upright posture, thoughtful leadership, a selfless act, a willingness to share, a warm gaze, a fun attitude, a motivated personality, an allure of libido — any display of genetic value can produce the attraction response in either sex, even ahead of physical attributes.

Beauty is fertility, and fertility is health. So many of today's magazines would flop if they simply told the biological truth: males value fertile females (and vice versa), and fertility depends chiefly on health. Therefore, if physical sex appeal is the goal, simply live an optimally healthy life and emphasize your fertility signals to become attractive. Unfortunately, most fertility signals are likely already determined. They depend largely on how healthy you were during your developmental years, since this is when most feminine traits are formed that signal fertility. However, it's never too late to improve your health, and fashion, clothing, and makeup are all things that can be utilized in the manipulation of fertility signals (wide hips, vibrant skin tone, broad shoulders, hint of facial hair, etc.).

Bond harder. The mechanisms that drive interpersonal bonding are talking, touching, sharing, cooperating, giving, playing, experiencing, and copulating. We owe it to ourselves to leverage these when building our tribes, and to employ them in the goal of bringing people even closer.

Resurrect group identity. Society necessitates many 'tribes'. In today's world, we form circles of friends around the structure of society. Your high school friends are a different circle than you college friends who are a different circle than your sports team. These circles will inevitably merge, but it's natural to grow them organically from the source as well, and to navigate them that way.

Meaningful relationships are more valuable. We may be hard-wired to chase sex and philander, but that doesn't mean that it's right or that it's best. Monogamy works great for those seeking a simple, deep primary pair bond. This should be cherished and embraced. Over time, people and the love they have for one another inevitably change, which may alter the relationship, but when it's done right, love grows.

Lastly, do things your way. Polyamory is natural to the ancestral environment but unnatural to the environment of civilization. In society, group identity, poly's mechanizing force, is dead. This places us in a complicated spot in modern society, lost but with many ways home. There are many different avenues to take with one's life in such a complex world of human sexuality. There is no need to feel anxiety or shame about your particular lifestyle just because society hasn't deemed it appropriate. Homosexuality, bisexuality, asexuality, polyamory, pansexuality, and many other forms of love, lust, and romance are totally legitimate lifestyles that work for many people. There's also no shame in being conventional. You can be a sheep. You can be a wolf. That's your choice.

Why are models skinny?

If men are supposed to prefer fertility signals, then why are models, our ambassadors of fashion and beauty, so darn frail? After all, many models are flat-chested, bony, and lack the curves of a fully formed woman. Some argue that models are supposed to look this way in order to better display clothing, others that fashion authorities purposely define the ideal female body as divergent from the norm. There are many possible explanations, but nevertheless: why are they the ones so commonly obsessed over, fawned at, and venerated by popular culture? One evolutionary explanation for the model's beauty lies directly in the model's lack of fertility signals — that is, her thin frame. While skinny models lack many physical fertility signals, they retain an important one: youth.

Women come of age biologically by their early teenage years, which provides some evolutionary insights into sexual maturity as nature defines it. Because women in their early teens are physically underdeveloped, they too lack the curves that are conventionally associated with female attractiveness, such as large breasts and wide hips. Models, in this way, mimic youth, which in turn signals fertility and genetic value, triggering our natural instincts about beauty.

Why do people kiss?

There's more to a kiss than you might think. For many women coming of age sexually, the kiss represents the first step in the formation of a relationship. In evolutionary terms, this is no small matter, since reproduction is at the heart of romantic relationships. Evolution would then predict that there is something more to a kiss than meets the eye. Consider prostitutes that will sleep with men but won't kiss them. Is there something more to this?

Like everything, the kiss itself was likely subject to evolution. Anthropologists posit that kissing likely started with food sharing between our pre-human ancestors. Once human, the kiss remained as a gesture of affection, but its role in relationships had taken on new biological importance.

The kiss is more than a simple gesture, because scientists have found that humans choose mates according to how they taste.[329] Behind this phenomenon is the major histocompatibility complex, which plays a major role in immunity. People tend to choose partners with a histocompatibility complex distinct from their own.[330] This bolsters their children's immune system by increasing their overall resistance to antigens.

Is Being Gay Natural?

An Evolutionary Analysis of Homosexuality

The things that are the most important to survival are the ones that ultimately become the most complex, varied, and divergent. Food, sex, sleep — these are areas in biology that are vastly complicated, endlessly mysterious, and hotly debated, as they will be for the foreseeable future. Homosexuality is among these mysterious aspects of human nature.

At first glance homosexuality is an evolutionary puzzle, because it seems to kill reproductive potential. After all, a man can't impregnate another man, and a woman can't impregnate another woman. However, much of the evidence points to an underlying genetic

[329] Kirschenbaum, Sheril. *The Science of Kissing*. Grand Central, 2011.

[330] Chaix R, Chen C, Donnelly P (2008). "Is Mate Choice in Humans MHC-Dependent?". *PLoS Genetics* 4 (9): e1000184.

component to homosexuality. For instance, there is a nearly consistent rate of homosexuality across human populations. David P. Barash, an evolutionary biologist at the University of Washington, writes,

> The concordance of homosexuality for adopted (hence genetically unrelated) siblings is lower than that for biological siblings, which in turn is lower than that for fraternal (non-identical) twins, which is lower than that for identical twins.[331]

The genetic component of homosexuality is contentious and puzzling, because it forces a hard question: If homosexuality is genetic, then how was it selected for? Obviously, gay people can't reproduce. Or can they?

Sexuality in many species is highly complex and mysterious. Gibbons practice group sex. Oysters can change gender and back again for mating. Male giraffes court other males more often than they do females.[332] Homosexual behavior has been observed in almost 1,500 species.[333] This means, of course, that homosexuality is natural in evolutionary terms. And human beings are no exception to the vast, complex world of biological sexuality. It is simply a natural phenomenon of evolution.

We don't fully understand the mystery of how homosexuality evolved, but we have plenty of good guesses. It may have been due to kin selection if homosexuals increased the reproductive success of their blood relatives; or, it may have been due to group selection if groups

---

[331] Barash, David P. "The Evolutionary Mystery of Homosexuality." The Chronicle of Higher Education. Retrieved from http://chronicle.com/article/The-Evolutionary-Mystery-of/135762/

[332] Coe M.J. (1967). "Necking" behavior in the giraffe. *Journal of Zoology* (London) 151 (3): 313–321.

[333] Bagemihl Bruce. *Biological Exuberance: Animal Homosexuality and Natural Diversity.* St. Martin's Press, 1999.

with some homosexuals fared better than groups of purely heterosexuals. It could also have been explained by the social prestige of homosexuality. Many cultures honor gayness, which in turn could bolster their biological reproduction with members of the opposite sex. Perhaps we have not yet discovered the genetic component that paired with a mechanistic counterpart, such as in the evolution of the sickle-cell gene. Or perhaps an antagonistic 'gay gene' in one sex may very well benefit the other sex. And lastly, perhaps homosexuality is not a trait itself that was selected for, but rather a byproduct of a mix of traits.[334] All of these possibilities hold water according to evolutionary theory.

So, we may not yet know *how* homosexuality evolved, but we do know that homosexuality *did* evolve. The implications to this are staggering. There are many manifestations of sexuality that are natural in evolutionary terms. This may fly in the face of conventional wisdom or propriety, especially if those wisdoms are informed by biased, bigoted, or religious perspectives, but it's the truth. I will say only that the social issues of our time must be decided on secular grounds. If those decisions are informed by science and reason, then our world will be better for it.

---

[334] Barash, David P. "The Evolutionary Mystery of Homosexuality." The Chronicle of Higher Education. Retrieved from http://chronicle.com/article/The-Evolutionary-Mystery-of/135762/

"Think of it: zillions and zillions of organisms running around, each under the hypnotic spell of a single truth, all these truths identical, and all logically incompatible with one another: 'My hereditary material is the most important material on earth; its survival justifies your frustration, pain, even death'. And you are one of the organisms, living your life in the thrall of a logical absurdity."

Robert Wright

science writer

CHAPTER 9

FOUNDATIONS FOR HUMAN VIRTUE AND THE EVOLUTION OF MORALITY

Just twelve thousand years ago there were sabre-tooth cats roaming the countryside. Giant short-faced bears and dire wolves hunted the same lands humans did, and at about that same time, at the turn of the Neolithic, they all disappeared. Everywhere humans go extinction follows.

This is no recent phenomenon, nor is it due to the spread of civilization. Before farming villages sprouted, humans had already reached most corners of the Earth as hunter-gatherers, and wherever they went, they reaped havoc on the land. Our ancestors turn out not to be the noble savages we thought them to be.

The great extinctions of the Stone Age were most likely at the hands of humans. The victims:

> ...giant bison, wild horse, short-faced bear, mammoth, mastodon, sabre-toothed cat, giant ground sloth and wild camel. By 8,000 years ago, eighty per cent of the large mammal genera in South America were also extinct — giant sloths, giant armadillos, giant guanacos, giant capybaras, anteaters the size of

horses.[335]

Extinction is the worst kind of death, because it represents the death of heritage, of lineage. This is a pattern of destruction that follows humans still. The first inhabitants of Hawaii killed off half of the bird species, many of which had not learned to be afraid of humans; across the pacific islands, over 2000 species of birds are now extinct due to human activities.[336] The fauna and megafauna of Australia, the Americas, and oceanic islands shared the same fate upon the arrival of humans. At Olsen-Chubbuck, an ancient bison kill site, Native Americans in Colorado hunted bison by stampeding them over a cliff. [337] They only claimed the best parts of a fraction of these slaughtered animals. This is a disturbing pattern of human nature, told by extinction, deforestation, and land degradation presumably since humans began walking the earth. Our penchant for taking from nature until it has nothing left to give may simply be a fundamental part of being human, one more thing to add to the list of dark truths.

But if humans are naturally greedy, wasteful, and destructive, why do we also find virtue, morality, decency, and goodness in our nature? The answer to this question begins, paradoxically, with the very selfishness to which this question alludes.

You Are No Complete Self-Altruist

The natural fascination with oneself is nothing new to contemporary society. It is an ancient obsession. We stared at ourselves in the reflections of still waters just as surely as we do now at mirrors and filtered social media photographs. There is no shame in that, lest taken too far. And as modern economics teaches us, not only is a self-centered view of the world natural —

---

[335] Ridley, Matt. *The Origins of Virtue.* Penguin, 1996. p 217.

[336] Steadman D (1995). Prehistoric Extinctions of Pacific Island Birds: Biodiversity Meets Zooarchaeology. *Science* 267: 1123-31.

[337] Wheat JB (1967). A Paleo-Indian Bison Kill. *Scientific American* 216 (1): 44–53.

it is practical. In fact, our entire capitalist economic system is built upon the idea that if we all act in our own self-interest, the invisible hand will guide the market toward mutual benefit and prosperity. We now understand what this metaphor actually stands for: comparative advantage, mutual benefit, division of labor, trade. Our first level of altruism, it would seem, is the generosity toward ourselves. As Gordon Gekko famously said, "Greed is good."

But it must be put to question that if we, in the biological sense, are acting on our 'selves's' behalf, then why are there so many points to the contrary? For instance, why do people sacrifice their lives for others? How is that kind of death good for our selfish selves? The truth is that we don't die for our 'selves' entirely. We balance that need with others, ultimately succumbing to the needs of our genes.

There are plenty of accounts of people dying for others, willingly giving up their lives for the greater good. They die to protect their family, their community, their country. Every war is rife with the lives of men who fought for themselves, for their loved ones, and for each other. The question is why. If we are indeed perfectly selfish, then why make the ultimate sacrifice, one that permanently and thoroughly disproves our selfishness? The evidence is glaringly obvious in the case against this notion of pure selfishness, instead pointing to a more complex picture of human behavior, one that was not fully understood until we discovered genes. Thereafter, the cynical view of a self-centered world crumbled around us. As Matt Ridley writes, "Biology softens economic lessons rather than hardens them."[338]

Immortal Genes

All organisms are said to be a collection of traits, but really what is meant is a collection of genes, since genes code for traits. And this is the mind-bender: it's your genes that are selfish, not you.[339] After all, 'you' in the

---

[338] Ridley, p 20.

[339] Dawkins, Richard. *The Selfish Gene*. Oxford University Press, 1990.

biological sense is merely a collection of genes, genes that are immortally competing and compromising with each other. The concept of 'you' is really only a handful of genes, such as the ones that lay out the architecture for consciousness. While this may seem to only affirm the dark truths we have covered, it also provides the only viable biological framework for understanding many of the phenomena seen in nature, including the good things in human behavior, like altruism.

Gene selection theory makes perfect mathematical sense. As one of the originators of the concept, George C. Williams, writes,

> ...the essence of genetical theory of natural selection is a statistical bias in the relative rates of survival of alternatives (genes, individuals, etc.). The effectiveness of such bias in producing adaptation is contingent on the maintenance of certain quantitative relationships among the operative factors.[340]

To rephrase: since genes are the currency of selection, then it must be the genes that are more successful that ultimately prosper. Thus, the genes that cause behavior that augments survival and reproduction must be the ones that make their way into an organism to stay, relative to other less successful genes and individuals.

In regard to altruism, one of the first questions that comes up is this: if the gene is the unit of selfishness, why does it align with other genes to compose the individual organism? Out of the irrationality of altruism emerges the rationality of alliance. From the first cell to the first organism to the first group to the first group of groups, the formation of an alliance with others has proven a competitive advantage in nature and fulfills an ancient pattern.

The first life on earth was atomistic and individual. Increasingly,

---

[340] Williams, George C. *Adaptation and Natural Selection.* Princeton University Press, 1966. pp. 22.

since then, it has coagulated. It has become a team game, not a contest of loners. By 3.5 billion years ago there were bacteria run by a thousand genes. Even then there was probably teamwork...By 500 million years ago there were complex bodies of animals comprising a billion cells...the biggest bodies have been getting bigger and bigger. The largest plants and animals that have ever lived on earth — the giant sequoia and the blue whale — are alive today...But already a new form of coagulation is occurring: social coagulation. By 100 million years ago there were complex colonies of ants run by teams of a million bodies or more and now they are among the most successful designs on the planet.[341]

The genes, in this case, have followed this historical pattern of coagulation. They have allied themselves with other useful genes in order to promote their own selfish interest: replication. The teams of genes that replicated the most successfully were the ones who proliferated at the expense of other genes and other teams of genes. You and I, as we know ourselves, are simply along for the ride. As Richard Dawkins once said, "We are survival machines — robot vehicles blindly programmed to preserve the selfish molecules known as genes. This is a truth which still fills me with astonishment."[342]

True Altruism is Ultimately Selfish

Altruism is seen in many species and it at first puzzled biologists, because altruism comes at a cost to the individual offering altruism, which would seem to decrease reproductive fitness. We tend to see altruism offered at different levels: to ourselves, our family, our friends and acquaintances, strangers, even pets and enemies. In the ancestral environment, these levels

---

[341] Ridley, pp. 14

[342] Dawkins, Richard. *The Selfish Gene*. Oxford University Press, 1976. Preface.

would most closely constitute our relatives, our group, and outsiders.

The most blatant example of altruism is our concern for family. Evolutionists struggled for a long time to reveal just why we tend to favor family. Parents go to great lengths and make huge sacrifices for their children, and vice versa. In fact, relatives in general care more about each other than non-relatives, so what explains this? What makes our relatives more special than others? And more importantly, what makes our relatives so special that we sacrifice for ourselves?

It's really only selfish gene theory that explains this behavior, because we share genes with our descendants, siblings, relatives, and ancestors. So right off the bat, we are more likely to ally with our families because they share our genes. In an evolutionary sense, their success is our success. Thomas Henry Huxley, Darwin's counterpart in Victorian England, believed that all altruism, rare in the dog-eat-dog world he believed in, could only be explained in the context of blood relatives.[343] Though Huxley didn't yet know the concept of genes, his prediction is surprisingly accurate. It's known as 'kin selection' now, where's helping one's relatives survive grants our genes an evolutionary advantage. But Huxley's contemporaries took issue with his position, because altruism is also seen outside the world of family. Indeed, we are altruistic even to pets, even more surely to friends and acquaintances, a phenomenon seen across many different species.

Enter the concept of 'group selection', the idea that a cohesive group will succeed over less cohesive groups. If cohesive groups are stronger than otherwise, then individual traits that forge cohesiveness will prevail. Even Darwin predicted this to be the case:

> ...he who was ready to sacrifice his life, as many a savage has been, rather than betray his comrades, would often leave no offspring to inherit his noble nature... a tribe including many members who...were always ready to give aid to each other and

---

[343] Dugatkin, Lee A (2007). Inclusive fitness theory from Darwin to Hamilton. *Anecdotal, Historical, and Critical Commentaries on Genetics* 176 (3): 1375-80.

sacrifice themselves for the common good, would be victorious over most other tribes; and this would be natural selection.[344]

Our evolved traits strengthen our groups, a fact which matches the pattern of coagulation that has surfaced since the beginning of time. Human beings still retain these evolved traits; they make us remarkably good at living in groups. We have language, relationships, emotions, conscience, etc. Together, these and other traits make us a winning team via cooperation, trade, and specialization. We are, after all, the sole survivors of several hominin species that simply couldn't make the grade. *Homo floresiensis, homo sapiens idaltu*, and *homo neanderthalensis* are all human species that are now extinct. We are social animals, and that sociality goes way deeper than many realize.

And here's where altruism starts to get murky, with acquaintances and strangers, even with pets and enemies. What was it about the ancestral environment that led to the rise of genes that supported this kind of behavior?

In Chapter 1, we discussed briefly the science of strategy known as game theory. It's a mathematical model that has been used a great deal in regard to evolutionary theory. One way that it has proved useful is in demonstrating the mathematical benefits of social interaction. In particular, game theory illuminates how a system based on egalitarianism, reciprocity, and cooperation can be mutually profitable from an evolutionary standpoint by mechanizing and rewarding altruistic behavior.

Weapons: the Technology of Egalitarianism

"I know not with what weapons World War III will be fought, but World War IV will be fought with sticks and stones."
Albert Einstein, hairstyle trend-setter

---

[344] Darwin, Charles. *The Descent of Man and Selection in Relation to Sex.* New York: Appleton. pp 163 and 166.

It may very well be that human beings played a major role in the extinction of many of the formidable species that dominated the earth. Of them, one of the most recent, and one of the most ironic, were the Neanderthal, because of how closely related they were to anatomically modern humans. They used tools, had culture, and were intelligent. They were also bigger and stronger. So why did they lose this unfortunate evolutionary struggle? What makes humans comparatively resilient if not their size and strength?

The two good answers are our brains and social ties. Humans are just a little bit smarter and a little bit more cohesive. And one of the things leading to this was the ubiquity of rather refined weaponry in the hands of humans.

The first tools were simple, more than likely used for accessing food. As weapons technology developed, they became more and more sophisticated and powerful. Their application to problems of hunting and survival forever changed human interactions, because they instituted an eternal Mexican standoff, forever changing the game of domination, violence, and coercion that characterizes so many mammalian species.

In a Mexican standoff, there are three opponents, rather than just two. In this scenario, it is granted that they each have weapons, making them each equally effective at an offensive. Strategically, you don't want to be first to shoot, because the person you did not shoot has the advantage of shooting you while you are busy shooting. So, not only does no one want to shoot first, but no one wants to shoot *period*. In evolutionary and tactical terms, this scenario helps us understand how weapons in a social setting helped mold a more egalitarian human culture, because size and strength, coercion and dominance, were no longer viable in a social hierarchy once weapons arrived.

Most other primates are notably hierarchical, and these chains-of-command see a great deal of violence and brutality. Many are surprised to learn that humans, compared to other animals, are relatively peaceful, cooperative, and egalitarian. This pleasantly surprising fact is true between sexes, among clan members, and throughout different ages. Could it be that weapons played a role in fueling this phenomenon?

Most people see weapons as a route to increasing violence. They picture weapons of mass destruction, horrific wars, and merciless dictators. Vladimir Lenin once said, "One man with a gun can control a hundred without one." But what about a hundred men, each with a gun, and all of them in the same clan? What happens then?

We know what happens because anthropologists have documented exactly this.

> Another important factor in this context is the access which all males have to weapons among the !Kung, Hadza, Mbuti and Batek. Hunting weapons are lethal not just for game animals but also for people. There are serious dangers in antagonising someone: he might choose simply to move away but if he feels a strong sense of grievance that his rights have been encroached upon he could respond with violence.[345]

Richard Lee has documented well the murders that occur among the !Kung.[346] And James Woodburn explains how the Hadza recognize "the hazard of being shot when asleep in camp at night or being ambushed when out hunting alone in the bush."[347] In this kind of environment, the pressures are high to keep the peace.

As the tactics of the Mexican standoff teach us, no one wants to be the first to put a target on their back. And the only way to do that, strategically, is to not shoot; or, in practical terms, it's best to not create enemies. Now scale that principle to a realistic level: dozens of clansmen, each with access to a primitive hatchet, club, dart, blunt edge, atlatl, or even heavy stone. All of these weapons spell certain doom for anyone with an enemy, no matter how

---

[345] Woodburn, J (1982). Egalitarian Societies. *Man* 17 (3): 431-51. pp. 436.

[346] Lee, Richard B. *The !Kung San: Men, Women, and Work in a Foraging Society.* Cambridge University Press, 1979. pp. 370-400

[347] Woodburn, J. *Minimal Politics: the Political Organization of the Hadza of North Tanzania.* Clarendon, 1979. pp. 252 [Quoted in Woodburn 1982]

big they are. An individual's size doesn't matter in the face of an alliance or against the element of surprise. And so strategy says, don't make enemies. If that's not the definition of peace, I don't know what is.

An old advertising slogan goes, "God made men, but Sam Colt made them equal." But it wasn't the invention of the six-shooter in 1836 that did it; weapons have been around as long as mankind. Over millions of years, the presence of weapons forever changed the direction of human evolution, steering us toward a more balanced social system, burning the principle of egalitarianism into the core of our conscience.

After all, the rules of the wild are unwritten. There are no rules but tacit ones, no laws but the laws of nature, nothing sovereign but the bonds of men and the sacred mystery of life itself. This is the only valid framework from which to understand the human obsession with freedom, independence, and equality. They are forever buried in the prism of human need, cardinal to our moral code.

The Myth of the Alpha Male

It's a trope in literature and popular culture, and it's seen nearly everywhere. The muscled, emotionless superhero, a lone wolf, guns blazing as he rides into glory, rescuing the damsel in distress and winning her heart, only to plant his seed and move on. It's an unfortunate consequence of the modern mythology of gender. Our young men are taught this false masculinity, one based on domination, violence, and emotionlessness. But perhaps most unfortunate, some men try to be this man when everything in our nature will make us despise him. And it's all because there is no such thing as a human alpha.

Domination, violence, and hierarchy among social animals are real things. They are seen in nature, in tribal agriculturalists, and in society today. Many social animals establish hierarchies that ultimately affect the health of each member of the group, depending on where they fall in the hierarchy. In many cases, dominance is the mechanism that establishes that hierarchy. It can take many forms, from the physical to the psychosocial, from fighting to tantalizing to tricking to teasing.[348]

Much of contemporary society is molded into hierarchy. It's the most popular form of corporate, political, and institutional organization. Power rises up the ranks, all the way to the top, in a natural human social formation. The presidents, the CEOs, the executives — conventional wisdom teaches us that these folks must be the contemporary versions of the tribal leaders and alphas. It's only natural that these exceptional few enjoy more resources, wield more power, and dictate nearly half the waking hours of their subordinates' lives, right?

Wrong. The truth is that while hierarchy and dominance are to some degree natural, today's hierarchies are not a natural human social formation. The truth is that today's organizations require hierarchy as a function of utility. It just so happens to be the most efficient way of getting things done. It elevates our economic efficiency, with a few exceptions that prove the rule. However, by no means does this match our natural inclinations; and further, these false social hierarchies only fuel discord with our evolved traits.

The myth of the alpha male is a story where status is won by domination, coercion, or force, directly or indirectly, violently or casually. It's a story where the lone victor, he against the world, bests his counterparts and hoards his winnings, often resources in the form of food, sex, or possessions. The alpha male is staunch and stolid, unyielding in his acquisition of power, careless of the well-being of others, and nescient of his own emotion. And it's all a lie, because there isn't a single thing natural about that.

Christopher Boehm is an anthropologist at the University of Southern California and has relentlessly studied and written about the phenomenon of egalitarianism in human culture. His findings are staggering. In the seminal book, *Hierarchy in the Forest*, Boehm outlines how natural tendencies toward domination and submission align with our emotions and moral framework to guide social hierarchy. Ryan Earley summarizes:

---

[348] Sapolsky, R (2005). The influence of social hierarchy on primate health. *Science* 308: 648-52.

...humans will forever experience a three-tiered 'psychological tug of war' where intrinsic tendencies toward dominance do battle with altruistic cultural and moral codes and with emotional resentment of domination.[349]

Boehm looks at our primate relatives, chimpanzees and bonobos, to draw assumptions about ancestral *Pan*, the shared predecessor of humans, bonobos, and chimpanzees. Leveraging characteristics of *Pan*, he details the rise of egalitarianism in our own species as an inevitable consequence of our developing brain, emerging moral code, and deepening social ties.[350]

The mechanism by which egalitarianism is achieved, Boehm argues, is by a system of 'reverse dominance', where subordinate members of the group keep dominant members in check by force, even killing them.[351] Boehm does not doubt that this is one way in which the human alpha male vanished from existence.

These subordinate rebellions may well have provided the evolutionary basis for the egalitarian social orders that typify the lifestyles of culturally modern hunter-gatherers and that in fact have continued to prevail among most tribal agriculturalists...

First, at the level of phenotype, we temporarily lost the alpha male role by becoming politically egalitarian... Second, at the level of genotype, we acquired a conscience (with a sense of shame) that made us moral. This changed the nature of our group life... [352]

---

[349] Earley, Ryan (2000). Balance of Power. *American Scientist* 88 (2):1.

[350] Boehm, Christopher. *Hierarchy in the Forest: the Evolution of Egalitarian Behavior.* Harvard University Press, 2001.

[351] Ladd KM (2011). Chimp murder in Mahale. [Web file] Retrieved from www.nomad-tanzania.com/blogs/greystoke-mahale/murder-in-mahale/

[352] Boehm, C (2012). Ancestral hierarchy and conflict. *Science* 336: 844-47.

Out of this ancestral environment, humans saw the rise of egalitarianism, a deep moral and emotional inclination toward preserving equality among members in a group.

And one of the defining features of this process, as Ryan Earley describes, is an "emotional resentment of domination." Humans, at the very core of their being, have an aversion to dominance.[353] They dislike alpha males so much that they are motivated to curb dominant behaviors, whether that be shunning, ostracizing, shaming, threatening, even murdering.[354] Boehme again on weapons:

> Subordinate resentment of domination, the ability to form large coalitions, and the capacity of such coalitions to dominate or eliminate a bully with their combined weaponry were sufficient to momentarily eliminate an alpha-type individual... In effect, egalitarianism could have arisen simply because humans became culturally able to form moral communities and were prone to rebel against dominant authority.[355]

Thus, with this breach in human evolutionary potential, we see the disappearance of the human alpha.

For humans today, these things spiral into layers of detail. We have even more tools at our disposal to curb dominant behaviors, and our level of intelligence means that we are even more sensitive to those behaviors. We are able to identify them according to nuanced levels of detail, whether that is someone interrupting you when you speak, contradicting what you say, or lightly making fun of you — even delicate social transgressions such as these can provoke their fair share of reciprocal vengeance. This is why overbearing personalities are so easily labeled as arrogant or threatening. Ironically,

---

[353] Fehr and Rockenbach (2004). Human altruism: economic, neural, and evolutionary perspectives. *Current Opinion in Neurobiology* 14 (6): 784-90.

[354] Boehm, Christopher. *Moral Origins: the Evolution of Virtue, Altruism, and Shame.* Basic, 2012.

[355] Boehm, Christopher. *Hierarchy in the Forest.* Harvard, 2001. pp 194-195.

personalities that seek respect from others by exhibiting dominant traits do so at the cost of the group's acceptance.

So strategy says, be good and fair, form alliances, stand up for yourself, but uphold others as equals, even in leadership. The ancient Chinese philosopher Lao Tzu said, "To lead people, walk behind them." I think that's the natural way to do it. But alphas are not limited only to males. Females also participate in this universal human instinct toward egalitarianism. So equal, in fact, that we can debate which sex evolution favored.

Questioning The Sexual Division of Labor

Man the hunter. It's a phrase burned into the cultural consciousness of our time. It ushers in conceptions of virility and male prowess. And, for some men, it provides an ancient justification for the sacred, central duty of manhood: to provide.

Males were the designated hunters of the tribe. Females helped out to some degree with small game and insects, securing their role in hunting, but it were the men who felled the mightiest beasts. In turn, many early anthropological ideas and popular ideas today point to this particular gender role leading to power in the social group, since food won hunting was a form of resource acquisition, much like working in today's corporate world is the fuel of patriarchy.

But in academia there lives a valid rebuttal to this idea, that the concept of 'man the hunter' is simply fueling patriarchal ideals by upholding the male role of resource acquisition in the ancestral environment. This rebuttal is summed up in The Gathering Hypothesis, which states that women played an important role in resource acquisition too, because women gathered significant amounts of food. Proponents of this hypothesis posit that 'man the hunter' glorifies male contributions while belittling female ones.[356]

Food was certainly a resource, but did hunting upset the balance of

---

[356] Buss, David. *Evolutionary Psychology: the New Science of the Mind.* Pearson, 2008.

power? We know that early human tribal formations were surprisingly egalitarian among its members, both among men[357] and between men and women.[358] Whether hunting back then was the game-changer, we can only guess. Of course, the feminist critique is highlighting the modern patriarchal view that honors male contribution by glorifying the gender role of hunting.

To unravel this assertion, consider the lion, where females do the hunting — and nearly everything else — leaving the males with little responsibility. After female lions have made a kill, sometimes the male takes the carcass, rarely sharing with the lionesses that did all the hard work. To many, this is clearly unfair that the females must take on an unequal burden of responsibility.

The lion represents a phenomenon in nature that can only truly be understood by evolution and the ethological pressures that govern the sexual division of labor. Lion prides usually have but one male, who protects the pride from other males. This leads females, who are more capable hunters than males, to work cooperatively in order to feed themselves and their cubs. Together, these facts and more dictate how and why females are the ones who do the dangerous work of bringing down prey.

In this objective context, is there really anything apparently glorious about hunting? Do we see the females or the males as the ones with power in this scenario? And what does that say about humans?

It appears that males in the lion kingdom have maintained a lazy kingship, one enabled by domination and monopoly. Their physical dominance allows them to take from the females. And with often only one male around, the females have little choice but to concede to his rule. In this environment, the females are the unlucky ones who are left to do the hard work of providing food for their pride in addition to carrying and rearing young, an unfortunate consequence of their evolutionary legacy.

In this light, hunting, as the anthro-feminists rightly point out, may not

---

[357] Boehm, Christopher. *Hierarchy in the Forest: the Evolution of Egalitarianism.* Harvard, 2001.

[358] Gowdy, John. *Limited Wants, Unlimited Means: a reader on Hunter-Gatherer Economics and the Environment.* Island Press, 1997.

simply be a glorified acquisition of resources, nor is it necessarily one that leads to power. Instead, is it possible that hunting can be seen as the lowly work performed by the less fortunate gender, a natural consequence of the species' evolved traits, environment, and social formation?

Human social formations are far different from those of lions. In humans, it is the males who hunt, despite their physical dominance. There are equal numbers of males and females within a tribe and tribes are egalitarian, providing a different dynamic for the sexual division of labor. If women primarily gather food and take care of the children, and men go off on long hunting journeys, then which gender seems to have the favorable position in this social formation? Can a favorable position in the social formation predict that gender's power?

Men evolved to hunt for various reasons. Physically, they are more capable. There are social and sexual rewards for providing food. Hunting is an arena where men compete for status and simultaneously cooperate for survival. Like lions, humans were required to hunt in order to survive.

Men today find joy and meaning in the hunt, but this does not discount the objective role of hunting in a natural social formation. Evolution teaches us that mechanisms must have arisen that supported males in hunting, such as the evolved traits of pride, status seeking, or a thirst for adventure, even glory. These traits, which are the basis for the meaning and joy that men today find in the hunt, only confirm the evolutionary perspective.

It's a valid question: are hunting males the lowly workhorses, or the glorious breadwinners we revere? Can objectivity exist in a realm so ancient, sacred, and primal? Perhaps the truth is somewhere in the middle.

The sexual division of labor calls out one of the most potent traits among males: sex drive. It is motivation for much of human behavior, and hunting is no exception.

...the Hadza men who are good at hunting enjoy considerable social rewards. Their success is envied by other men and, perhaps more important, admired by the women. Good hunters, to put it bluntly, have more extramarital affairs. This is not confined to the Hadza. It applies to the Ache, the Yanomamo and other South American tribes; it is probably universal and it is no secret.[359]

Matt Ridley explains how men across tribal cultures tend to irrationally prefer hunting big prey. Small prey is easier and safer to procure, a more efficient use of time in order to feed oneself and one's family. In other words, going after small prey means less work for more food. But big prey differs from small prey in that it can be shared with the entire tribe, boosting one's status and access to mates, and this is exactly what is seen: men go after the big prey that can be shared with others in order to reap the social and sexual rewards.

This sheds light on the nature of male behavior because it explains male motivation in regard to the labor of hunting. Male sex drive is the driving force behind their willingness to do great feats for others, a cornerstone of their altruistic behavior. Moreover, sex drive is the mechanism by which males are biologically coerced into disproportionate acts of arduous labor and irrational acts of danger, risking their health, their bodies, and even their lives for the reward of reproduction. How glorious does hunting seem in this pathetic context? (I use the word pathetic, in this case, to connote inferiority in the sexual division of labor and the pathology therein, arising as social ills specific to males.)

It's also likely that the glory of hunting (or more specifically, the honorable act of provision) is a cultural meme, an analogue to the ethological necessity of resource acquisition and reproduction. It's a meme that honors male provision simply out of the prodigious investment that males have poured into the provision system, as well as the advantages that women reap from this system. Most feminists don't complain about free drinks from men at bars, nor the acts of chivalry. Feminists rally for more female doctors and politicians but do not seem to rally for more female coal miners and farm hands. Only evolution and the ethological pressures that govern the balance

---

[359] Ridley, p 112.

of power make sense of this.

The provision system's natural consequences — sex, reproduction, love, respect, affection, and status — are so central to human yearning that no man would forfeit his place at the table, even despite its objective purpose: to define ancestral men as worker bees. This may indicate why, even today, hunting and its traditionally modern counterpart, labor in the workplace, are seen as inherently male virtues. And despite this rather unfortunate ethological turnout for males, the sexes were strikingly egalitarian, especially as compared to other mammals. But all that changed with the rise of civilization.

When early civilization arose, men were at a natural advantage. This new system was based on goods and services, work and labor. Men, more physically capable, became useful to systems of power, whether it be through the production of farm goods or the engagement of war. This and many other factors upset the natural balance of power among the sexes, which prior to this was significantly more egalitarian. Culture only further fueled the division of labor, confining women to a life of domesticity, cut off from the new financial and economic power that would conquer the world.

When you marry evolution to this history, the entire background of feminism makes more sense and to a certain degree is legitimated. The very fuel by which it burns in the hearts of women and men today is rooted in the egalitarianism of an ancient moral code that struggles to make sense of the structure of society.

Women had to fight the status quo over centuries to win the right to toil behind desks and to rise the ranks of male hierarchies, while every man born is simply expected to embrace his societal duty, somehow impotent if he does not. Interestingly, feminism can generally be seen as the modern movement to reclaim the woman's status in the natural human social formation, one based on egalitarianism and equity in the balance of power. Ironically, in the environment of civilization, they must do so by entering the traditional and historical domain of men, attaining power and status as worker bees, at once shunning the domestic sphere so ancient to female culture and adopting labor as their own source of power. All out of the necessity of the environment.

The dynamics of civilization naturally favored male contribution, leading to a disproportionate rise in male power. In early civilization, the exploits that gained power favored the physical, giving men a natural advantage in the context of civilization for winning power. It took a long time for humans to achieve the societal stability and technological advancement that paved the way for women to reclaim their equality, a fight that still rages on today. It is a struggle that is noble, inevitable, and justifiable in the light of evolution, even though the movement itself generally shuns evolutionary theory and the contributions it can make to the cause.

Reciprocity

Many people are drawn to the idea of karma. They see that actions tend to form a balance, that deeds have an equalizing cause and effect. In other words, what goes around comes around. However, many people aren't aware that these sentiments are rooted in our evolutionary past, and they are one more aspect of human virtue.

Reciprocity describes the phenomenon of giving and taking. As many philosophies have noted, this tends to occur in an endless cycle, a back and forth. The background of reciprocity makes sense from an evolutionary perspective even at a superficial level, and it's observed in other social animals, which confirms its utility in nature. We already covered the potential sexual rewards for men that share, so what is it about reciprocity that makes it a viable strategy for survival, outside of the sexual realm?

Reciprocity is a form of social insurance that is necessitated by the nature of food acquisition. In the wild, food is at times scarce. Hunters and gatherers often return from their pursuits empty-handed simply based on the availability of food and the chances for success. Given this environment, it's sensible that when one has procured more than they can consume, that they share it with others in good faith that the favor will one day be returned. It was in this environment that our moral compass for reciprocating and honoring generous acts first appeared.

The growing human brain took our morality into uncharted territory, because it advanced the reciprocal act into an unprecedented achievement: explicit trade. Once goods were readily available, it set the framework for exchange, cooperation, and economy — all of which would eventually become a keystone of our species. This helps to answer an important question: how and why did we rise above the dog-eat-dog world of the wild and learn compassion, empathy, and temperance toward strangers?

Cooperation

People often recognize the incredible cultural diversity that exists in our world, across races, nations, cultures, and subcultures. However, most often do not recognize the degree of conformity that appears within these units of culture. Consider the totally veiled women of the middle East contrasted with the nudists of Germany. These are whole sub-cultures that are on polar ends of the spectrum from each other, displaying the rich diversity of the world.

Yet, within these cultures, something more interesting is happening, because within the different factions is a powerful driving force: conformity. Those within these groups are driven to behave in ways that align with the others in complementary ways, often through imitation. The fascinating thing about conformity is its prevalence in nature. Conformity can be seen in a flock of birds changing direction in flight. It can be seen in a school of fish evading a predator. And just like these, conformity in human behavior can be seen as a natural impulse.

Conformity is an ancient way of crowdsourcing information. As Matt Ridley explains,

> If others are unanimous in their choice, then the person may ignore his or her own opinion in favour of the herd's. This is not a weak or foolish thing to do. After all, other people's behaviour is a useful source of accumulated information. Why

trust your own fallible reasoning powers when you can take the temperature of thousands of people's views?[360]

Seen in this light, it makes sense why evolution would bestowed upon us a natural tendency to do as others do. The bird that does not flock may miss a mating opportunity. The fish that does not school may be exposed to a predator. Humans are no different, right?

Actually, we are, because humans are smart enough to know better. We can see the dark side of conformity, the foolishness of fads and the falsity of conventions. All conventions are merely temporarily venerated ideas. The flock of birds veer direction with little respect for rational decision making or optimization of strategy. So when humans make this mistake, it's surprising but understandable given its nature. Humans see fads, trends, and norms, some of which can be as ridiculous as the pet rock or as sacred as any conventional wisdom: *skim milk for strong bones!* The problem, as history shows us, is that these conventional wisdoms can commit bad logic. Worse still, they can lead to flash judgments, xenophobia, and bigotry.

Conformity is important for other reasons too, though. For humans, it's vitally important that others can be trusted. After all, trust is the currency of social interaction.

> Trust is as vital a form of social capital as money is a form of actual capital...Trust, like money, can be lent ('I trust you because I trust the person who told me he trusts you'), and can be risked, hoarded or squandered. It pays dividends in the currency of more trust.[361]

One way trust is established with others is in their ability to conform. Conformity is almost by definition a willingness to cooperate with others, to mimic their values and customs, a sign of their trustworthiness. Men are

---

expected to have a fresh short haircut for job interviews just as women are expected to wear skirts, dresses, or whatever is the fashion of the time. Conformity can even be a predictor of social cohesion. Big cities tend to have rebellious individualizing fashions while small towns can be starkly homogenous. Those who do not conform may face social stigma or even exile.

This brings us to an inviolable human trait, one that is the backbone of our strength as social animals: the natural tendency to cooperate. Rather advanced forms of cooperation are seen in many mammals,[362] but humans take the cake on this one. Our collaborative spirit has paved the way for amazing achievements. All of our evolved architecture in regard to morality leads us to be a highly cooperative species. Our evolved moral architecture is the framework for capitalism, trade, and comparative advantage. At least in part, it is responsible for opening the floodgates of human potential.

And finally, we draw toward an end in this world of human virtue. We see that it is egalitarianism and reciprocity, our sense of fairness and justice molded by the ancestral environment, that paints a deeper understanding of what it means to be human and how we got to where we are today. It was not simply the coercive hands of civilization that wrangled our human nature into submission, but rather human nature itself that complemented and fueled many of the innovations of civilization: democracy, capitalism, free trade, the nation-state. These are all the seemingly inevitable manifestations of our evolved morality — they make perfect sense given the natural history of our species.

What Evolution Says About God

Look around you. The signs are everywhere. There are churches and prayers and symbols and rituals and books and movies, a plethoric list of

---

[362] de Waal, Frans (2011). Frans de Waal: Moral Behavior in Animals. [Video file] Retrieved from http://www.ted.com/talks/frans_de_waal_do_animals_have_morals.html

things with religious origins. About half of America is religious in strict terms and the vast majority of the world is religious in loose terms. There are countless religions. Even recent ones grow rapidly. This may sound disingenuous, but in some ways evolution legitimizes religion, because evolution places religion into that sacred category of human need.

Perhaps this story starts with one of the central and defining characteristics of our species: human neoteny. Over evolutionary time, humans were subject to this phenomenon, neoteny, where adults retained characteristics that were previously seen only in the young. Hairlessness, upright spines, and playful attitudes have characterized the early development of primates far longer than they have characterized the behavior of humans. Our species simply evolved to retain these traits, expressing them into maturity, and they ultimately came to define our species. As geneticist Raymond St. Leger said, "Adult humans, in many ways, are essentially baby chimps."

We all understand the call of a child, whether it's the coy innocence of its face or the blaring resonance of its wail. We adore how much the baby needs us, that, to this delicate creature, we are strong and powerful and good and caring. This baby calls for support, for help, for love, for attention. It wants to be heard, consoled, and connected to the world around it. But this baby will grow up, and when it does its call for the love and support of an adult will echo forever in its consciousness. This is a consequence of neoteny. In Mark 10:14-15: "Jesus said to them, Let the little children come to me, and do not hinder them for the kingdom of God belongs to such as these. Truly, I tell you, anyone who will not receive the kingdom of God like a little child will never enter it." Is it any wonder that "Father" is so often used in this capacity?

There is nothing wrong with bearing the traits of a juvenile. It was neoteny that gave adults the gift of play, the powerful engine of creativity, and what led to bipedalism. The need to believe in God was simply installed upon our moral architecture long before we became *Homo sapiens*, creating the platform for the vast world of religion that we see today. How else can we explain the ubiquity of religious tomes in human culture? Are we to believe that these are simply a reflection of human invention? Clearly there is something instinctive to faith, something that fulfills a need deeper than curiosity.

> Religion is so natural to humanity that it seems to be part of human nature, as if a propensity for belief in the supernatural were genetically engraved in the human mind, and expressed as spontaneously as the ability to appreciate music or to learn one's native language.[363]

In *The Faith Instinct*, Nicholas Wade explores the universality of religion and its possible place in prehistory, ultimately concluding that religion evolved to help groups cohere.

Hard atheists and anti-theists are averse to this idea because they fear it will legitimize the tyranny of religious institutions, allowing them to further plunder scientific thought, spread false ideals, and fuel political bigotry. However, the faith instinct also highlights the good in religious practice: building community, nurturing optimism, relieving anxiety, promoting security in various forms, and fulfilling our innate need to rely on something stronger and bigger than we are. Perhaps in this light we can redefine the value and meaning of God, the church, and the self.

It is true to some degree that religion vies with evolution, logic, and science. Religion retains weak standards of evidence and can be dangerously manipulated for political purposes. One need only look at the current gay rights struggle to see bigotry and hate under the facade of religion. There are many ways that religion has detracted from human potential, but there are many ways that religion has advanced human potential. It should be the goal of religion to embrace evolution, science, and logic, and to exist in the gaps of human understanding, beyond the reach of science, promoting a complementary spirituality instead of a competing one. Religion manifests itself out of human need as a form of security in the mystery of death. It will

---

[363] Wade, Nicholas. *The Faith Instinct.* Penguin, 2009. p 5.

never disappear entirely. It is itself subject to its own kind of evolution. Religion adapts to the ideals and values of the culture that contains it. Consider churches 50 years ago that justified racism with God's word. It's important to note that racism was not fueled by God's word per se — it was fueled by racist people but placed in God's name to give their messages authority, an important distinction that parallels many of the controversial issues today. This was a reflection of secular bigotry in the name of religion, not simply religious bigotry. Today, this level of racism is almost unheard of, due to the shift in values of American culture. As the cultural climate changed in regard to race relations, the churches too adapted to the environment. The average church evolved according to the pressures of its environment; those that did not simply perished, went extinct — this is the truth of evolution. And it is one more important reason why we have seen the vast majority of hateful messages disappear over the last 50 years.

Bigotry in the name of the bible or any other sacred text is still a problem today for new frontiers of human progress and probably always will be due to the nature of social change and religious change. In another 50 years, churches will be more progressive, because the people will be too. After all, a church cannot survive without its congregation. In light of the evolution of religion, religious ideals and values historically trail the ideals and values of a society, but they adapt in parallel; thus, the eternal socio-political battle rages on.

Strategies in Virtue and Morality

Make a habit of appropriately thinking of others. Human goodness is, by definition, the greater good of the group. This is often at the expense of the individual. Conversely, selfishness is the definition of evil.

Respect the many planes of egalitarianism. Benign hierarchy is to some degree natural; humans form a meritocracy, where roles are based on ability. However, domination and coercion are easily detected and put to rest when possible, almost universally, based on human instincts. Liberty and personal autonomy are granted by nature, and egalitarianism is a human craving even within this meritocracy. Seeing how society upsets this balance may help us rectify the many wrongs of inequality among/between sexes, genders, races, classes, sexualities, ages, abilities, etc.

Uphold hope and faith without delusion. Humans are naturally optimistic. Our evolved psychologies yearn for hope and faith in order to assuage our insecurities, which were enabled by our big brains, an unfortunate cost of that power. Some faiths, like Buddhism, are friendly to science and can benefit well-being.

Reciprocate and cooperate with others. Ritual and religion can be seen as a means of upholding cultural conformity and therefore group cohesion, because one's willingness to conform signals trustworthiness. Rebellious individuality, on the other hand, while valuable, may have social costs if taken too far. Even the most generous people expect reciprocity.

"Death is the mother of beauty."

Wallace Stevens

American poet

CHAPTER 10

SUSTAINABILITY AND THE LESSONS OF ECOLOGY

The idea that man can control nature is a common theme in science fiction. Our storytellers dream of a future where we can improve Earth's climate, achieve sustainability, or even bring life to a barren world. It's an idea that is commonly explored in movies, books, and works of fiction, perhaps harboring some deep human yearning to one day wield the power to manipulate the laws of nature, to play god not only to solve our worldly problems but also to continue our colonial destiny into space, perhaps even one day populating Mars. The popular science fiction crowd seems to enjoy ideas like these, but many of them may be surprised to find that humans have already, to some degree, achieved this fiction. And it starts with Darwin's best-kept secret.

Ascension Island was a lifeless volcanic rock when young Charles Darwin, at the time an ambitious adventurer, first walked its shores. Today, it has transformed into a lush tropical landscape. A "cloud forest," as reported by the BBC. And a surprisingly simple plan made it possible.

Darwin was good friends with botanist Joseph Hooker, and when they arrived to Ascension in 1843, they observed a dry, desolate place. No fresh water. No trees. It barely supported life and the scant rains that fell quickly evaporated away. The island was victim to anhydrous trade winds blowing from South Africa that left this rock, swimming half an ocean from anywhere, utterly desiccated. But there was hope in Darwin's mind, so he and his dear friend Hooker hatched a plan.

At Darwin's encouragement, Hooker arranged, through an uncle at Kew Gardens, for trees to be transported to Ascension. The simplicity of this plan was its genius, because it concentrated on the most important part of an ecology, the canvas of life itself, the soil. As the plan went, "Trees would capture more rain, reduce evaporation, and create rich, loamy soils."[364] Starting in 1950, the island received shipments of trees, a mix of species from similar climates. Within thirty years, eucalyptus, Norfolk pine, bamboo, and banana were proliferating in what was to become the beginning of this new Eden.

Today, Ascension's peak is a lush forest. It represents a major victory for the future of terraforming. It stands as an historical relic to the modern farm movement, one that also leverages the lessons of ecology in order to bolster the strength of an ecosystem. This powerful idea is being applied by people today in a way that serves a greater purpose for our planet.

As they say, 'Life is good'. There's something to this, terraforming, the process of modifying an environment. It surfaces regularly in pop art and science. The question is, why? What's the appeal? Is it interesting only as a futuristic possibility? Does it echo a human longing to dominate nature? Perhaps these and other things. But deep down we all know and understand, from the very cores of our being, that protecting life, promoting life, and participating with life are all profoundly good things. Life is precious. This is something that we all know deep down to be true. The ability to play god, to turn a barren landscape into something that can sustain life, ignites a part of our deeper consciousness and morality that adores the idea. It is, perhaps, the

---

[364] Falcon-Lang, Howard (2010). "Charles Darwin's ecological experiment on Ascension Isle." *BBC News* [Web file] Retrieved from http://www.bbc.co.uk/news/science-environment-11137903.

greatest good of all. And it's something that is intrinsic to any discussion about sustainability.

The Lessons of Ecology

'Overpopulation' is a word that gets thrown around a lot in relation to ecology. Deer are a great example. Anywhere humans go, other apex predators are killed off or pushed out. The wolves and bear that populated the woods, prairies, and shores are, in most of North America, no longer present, or at least not so in significant numbers. That means that the predators keeping the deer population in check are no longer doing so, and the deer run riot.

Deer are lovely animals. Who didn't grow up loving Bambi? We are all fans of adorable creatures; we can't help but root for their growing population. It hits home for many of us, and it's hard to separate our affection for one animal with the reality of their ecological harm. As Ted Williams writes,

> In the southern part of the Lake Gaillard watershed, where we started out, there were now about 100 deer per square mile; in this kind of habitat you start seeing damage at about 15. In a 10-year experiment, the U.S. Forest Service found that at more than 20 deer per square mile you lose your eastern wood pewees, indigo buntings, least flycatchers, yellow-billed cuckoos, and cerulean warblers . At 38 deer per square mile you lose eastern phoebes and even robins. Ground nesters like ovenbirds, grouse, woodcock, whippoorwills, and wild turkeys can nest in ferns, which deer scorn, but these birds, too, are vastly reduced, because they need thick cover.[365]

---

[365] Williams, Ted. "Wanted: More Hunters." *Audubon Magazine.* [Web file] Retrieved from http://archive.audubonmagazine.org/incite/incite0203.html

Deer, as harmless as they seem, have the power to destroy an environment — the power to render a habitat uninhabitable. For the animals within that habitat, that spells extinction.

Of course, this phenomenon appears only without the presence of natural predators. The disappearance of predators is fully explained by the presence of the humans that drove them out, a practice our species has been refining for at least 12,000 years, from the mountains lions to the saber-tooth and beyond.[366] And it's something that our cultural ethos is almost comfortable with. But now there are no more predators to push out.

Predation is the ecological mechanism by which grazing animal populations are kept sustainable, balanced with the rest of the environment in a cycle of life that is itself literally endless. In this way, the deer need cougars just as much as the cougars need them. In a populated or residential area, where humans don't or can't normally hunt, these animals have nothing to limit their population.

Without a natural predator to limit their numbers, deer will destroy the flora that countless creatures, animals, and birds rely on. And they will write their own death sentence. Ted Williams again:

> That's what I saw in the early 1980s on the Crane Estate, 30 miles north of Boston, where roughly 400 white-tailed deer — 340 more than carrying capacity — had denuded 2,000 acres. There wasn't a scrap of green to the height of a saddle horn. One of the last undeveloped barrier-beach complexes in the East had been shorn of native plants. Dunes were blowing away. The property, owned by the Trustees of Reservations, was supposed to be a wildlife refuge, yet the deer had eliminated wildlife that rear young and/or find cover in mid-level vegetation. Each

---

[366] Haynes, Gary. "Did Humans Cause the Late Pleistocene-Early Holocene Mammalian Extinctions in South America?" *American Megafaunal Extinctions at the End of the Pleistocene.* Springer, 2009. p 139

winter most of the fawns died because they couldn't reach the browse line. In their weakened condition adults were being eaten from the outside in by dogs and from the inside out by parasites. Their skin stretched across their ribs like cloth...

The deer in this habitat literally ate themselves into oblivion. They ate until the flora was gone. They ate until the soil turned to dust and scattered in the wind. As Lierre Keith summarizes, "Without predators, the land dies." This is the simple ecological truth, a law of nature.

Another truth: humans are apex predators. Perhaps that's hard to swallow, but the fact remains that our ancestors have hunted animals since the dawn of our species and scavenged animals for about a million years before the first humans were born.[367] *Three and a half million years of documented animal consumption.* Indeed, hunting was our ancestor's contribution to the natural environment. Michael Pollan writes,

> Human hunting...literally helped form the American Plains bison, which...changed both physically and behaviorally after the arrival of the Indians.[368]

Lierre Keith expands on Pollan's idea in her book, *The Vegetarian Myth,*

> *And large ruminants changed humans just as surely as we changed them* [her emphasis]. The high-quality proteins and fats, especially the nutrient-dense organ meats, meant our digestive systems could shrink and our brains could grow. The megafauna of the prehistoric world, the aurochs and antelopes and mammoths, literally made us human. There is a reason they

---

[367] Lovett, Richard. "Butchering dinner 3.4 million years ago." *Nature.* [Web file] Retrieved from http://www.nature.com/news/2010/100811/full/news.2010.399.htmlhttp://www.nature.com/news/2010/100811/full/news.2010.399.html

[368] Pollan, Michael. *The Omnivores Dilemma.* Penguin, 2006. p 322

were our first, endless art project.[369]

The relationship between predator and prey is a mutually beneficial one, because predator and prey rely on each other as players within a dynamic, balanced ecology. Without balance, the ecology goes awry. Some of the most important questions about sustainability are answered only by the field of ecology, which is itself one of the first disciplines to fully trust the science of evolution. Natural ecologies are, by their very definition, sustainable. It is the field of ecology that illuminates the relationships that each life form has with each other life form and the relationship that each life form has with its environment. Inherent to those relationships is the heart of what defines sustainability.

Current models of sustainability take a measured approach to the discussion, starting from where we are now rather than starting with the reality of nature. Like any complex discipline, the topic of sustainability sees a great deal of discord among its experts. Some cry warnings of doomsday. 'It's already too late. Humans are overpopulated, and there is no hope other than diminishing our population and radically fighting the forces of destruction'. Others sing the hope of technology and the optimism of human progress. 'We can expect our agricultural methods to gain efficiency. Humans will make advancements on minimizing waste, utilizing clean energy, and living within their ecological means. Who knows what advancements will come in the future?' How do we make sense of this?

Institutionalized environmentalism in politics and academia ends up somewhere in the middle, both declaring the drastic need for improving the agricultural system, but working within the framework of political and socio-economic conventions to do so. In a 2010 paper, experts call for promising areas of exploration:

What people are talking about today, both in the private and

---

[369] Keith, Lierre. *The Vegetarian Myth: Food, Justice, and Sustainability*. Flashpoint, 2009. p 28

public research sectors, is the use and improvement of conventional and molecular breeding, as well as molecular genetic modification (GM), to adapt our existing food crops to increasing temperatures, decreased water availability in some places and flooding in others, rising salinity, and changing pathogen and insect threats. Another important goal of such research is increasing crops' nitrogen uptake and use efficiency, because nitrogenous compounds in fertilizers are major contributors to waterway eutrophication and greenhouse gas emissions.[370]

The authors of this paper, like anyone facing the reality of environmental destruction, acknowledge the growing need for changing the agricultural system. In fact, they lay out a laundry list of challenges. But the "radical" changes they propose only double-down, to use a gambling term, on the very system that has led us to modern food production challenges, hoping biotechnology, precision management, and government intervention will solve the crises of the future. The same crises this system helped to create.

The profit-maximizing agro-industrial complex scrambles for future technological solutions, pouring money into this system of patentable food technology with the hope that it reaps rewards down the line, disregarding ecological consequences and dangers to human health. What's wrong with this route? A 2013 paper appearing in *Agronomy for Sustainable Development* covers two obstacles,

> The first obstacle is the claim that genetically modified crops are necessary if we are to secure food production within the next decades. This claim has no scientific support, but is rather a reflection of corporate interests. The second obstacle is the resultant shortage of research funds for agrobiodiversity

[370] Fedoroff et al (2010). Radically Rethinking Agriculture for the 21st Century. *Science* 327(5967): 833-834.

solutions in comparison with funding for research in genetic modification of crops. Favoring biodiversity does not exclude any future biotechnological contributions, but favoring biotechnology threatens future biodiversity resources. An objective review of current knowledge places GM crops far down the list of potential solutions in the coming decades.[371]

Institutional environmentalists seek sustainability within an inherently unsustainable model, the irony of which is that we have already found sustainability. And it has been operating on this planet for eons. It was here before we were. Again: natural ecologies are, by definition, sustainable. They have been, and will be, sustainable since the beginning of time and into the future as we know it. They will do so according to natural laws, a give and take by each member of an ecosystem that is immersed in chaos, beauty, and balance.

The Scourge of Agriculture

Natural ecologies are at odds with — and losing to — conventional methods of food production. Almost all agriculture across the world is grown with grains, legumes, and tubers in the form of annual monocrops. The staples are wheat, rice, soy, corn, and potatoes. They account for roughly half of all calories that humans consume, and they have played a pivotal role in the ballooning of the population since the industrial revolution.

The rise of agriculture has severely impacted local ecologies around the globe. In the words of environmental physicist Dr. Daniel Hillel,

The evolution of agriculture left an ever-stronger imprint on the land in many regions. The vegetation, animal populations,

---

[371] Jacobsen et al (2013). Feeding the world: genetically modified crops versus agricultural diversity. *Agronomy for Sustainable Development* [ePub]. Retrieved from http://link.springer.com/article/10.1007/s13593-013-0138-9

slopes, valleys, and soil cover of land units were radically altered... with the result that the practice of farming there could not be sustained in the long run.[372]

The negligent use of the land by agriculturalists is what led to the Dust Bowl of the Southern Great Plains in the 1930s, forcing entire farming communities to find new soils. Today, similar challenges are seen in the African Sahel, the Aral Sea Basin of Central Asia, the Murray-Darling Basin of Australia, and the San Joaquin Valley of California.[373] Hillel comments,

> ...human exploitation of the land began early in history, we find disturbing examples of once-thriving regions reduced to desolation by human-induced degradation... The same anthropogenic processes that began in the early history of civilization have continued ever since, on a more extensive scale.[374]

There are also the tropics, too hot to support an ecology without rainforests, yet agricultural development is the leading cause of deforestation.[375] Clearing forests, turning fecund soils into dust, and destroying the natural habitat of countless living things, spelling death for niche species. Do I really need to explain why that's unsustainable?

As the population rises, there is more pressure on these crops to keep people fed, which is why big companies and researchers are seeking ways to maximize crop yields and solve all the challenges contained therein: feeding 9 billion people by 2050 using less water, less fertilizer, and fewer pesticides.[376]

---

[372] Hillel, Daniel. "Soil in the History of Civilization." *Soil in the Environment: Crucible of Terrestrial Life.* Elsevier, 2008. p 12

[373] Hillel, p 13.

[374] Hillel, p 13.

[375] World Bank. "Adaptation and Mitigation of Climate Change in Agriculture." *World Development Report 2008: Agriculture for Development.* p 201.

[376] Nature News Feature (2010). Food: the growing problem. *Nature* 466: 546-547.

And maybe — just maybe — they'll do so without using more land, as Britain's Royal Society has advised.[377] Even if the engines of agriculture eventually achieve the asymptotic climb in efficiency that many, including myself, believe they will, agricultural monocropping still comes at great cost to the environment.

Worst of all, monocrops require 'biotic cleansing'. Quite literally, this means wiping out all forms of life in order to lay down crops and then engaging in biochemical warfare to keep them at bay; animals, pests, and bacteria are simply not allowed to coexist. Lierre Keith describes this poignantly:

> And agriculture isn't quite a war because the forests and wetlands and prairies, the rain, the soil, the air, can't fight back. Agriculture is really more like ethnic cleansing, wiping out the indigenous dwellers so the invaders can take the land. It's biotic cleansing, biocide ... It is not non-violent. It is not sustainable. And every bite of food is laden with death... There is no place left for the buffalo to roam. There's only corn, wheat, and soy. About the only animals that escaped the biotic cleansing of the agriculturalists are small animals like mice and rabbits, and billions of them are killed by the harvesting equipment every year. Unless you're out there with a scythe, don't forget to add them to the death toll of your vegetarian meal. They count, and they died for your dinner... Soil, species, rivers. That's the death in your food. Agriculture is carnivorous: what it eats is ecosystems, and it swallows them whole.[378]

From it's very foundations, agriculture is unsustainable — yet everything

---

[377] The Royal Society (2009). Reaping the Benefits: Science and the Sustainable Intensification of Global Agriculture. [PDF web file] Retrieved from http://royalsociety.org/policy/publications/2009/reaping-benefits/

[378] Keith, Lierre. The Vegetarian Myth. Flashpoint, 2009. pp 37, 40, 42.

business and government seem to be doing to achieve sustainability operate within this agricultural paradigm, economically feasible though it may be, as if there are no other options. They'll fertilize the soil with fossil fuels and disturb the free market with subsidies and then wonder why malnutrition, starvation, and waste are huge global problems.

Monocrops also deplete topsoil, the most important part of an ecology. Soil is living matter that is itself grown over years, even decades, providing nutrients and lifeblood to flora and fauna alike — it is the keystone of an ecology. In an ecosystem, soil is naturally replenished; in monocropping, it is turned to dust or barely kept alive with fossil fuels, taking years and years to return to fertility. By one account, today's crops are "reducing soil productivity 18 times faster than it takes to rebuild it."[379] Additionally, somewhere from two-thirds and up to 95% of our land grains are grown to support industrial livestock[380] — a system that has hijacked almost all of the American prairie and 99% of Canada's stable organic matter called humus.[381] After consecutive years of cropping, nutrients in the topsoil are depleted,[382] which adversely affects both the nutrition for the growing plant, and for the end user: you.[383]

Soil is a precious and finite resource. Wes Jackson and Wendell Berry chime in for the *New York Times*:

> ...damage has been done in the long run...by various degradations resulting from industrial procedures and technologies alien to both agriculture and nature. Soil that is used and abused in this way is as nonrenewable as (and far more valuable than) oil. Unlike oil, it has no technological substitute

[379] Roslin, Alex (2008). "Monocrops bring food crisis." *Straight*. [Web file] Retrieved from http://www.straight.com/news/monocrops-bring-food-crisis.

[380] Pojman, Paul. *Food Ethics*. Cengage Learning, 2011. p 154.

[381] Mollison, Bill. *Permaculture: A Designer's Manual*. Tagari, 1988. p 205.

[382] Miller and Spoolman. *Sustaining the Earth*. Cengage Learning, 2008. p 154.

[383] Policy Statement (2007). Toward a Healthy, Sustainable Food System. *American Public Health Association*. [Web file] Retrieved from http://www.apha.org/advocacy/policy/policysearch/default.htm?id=1361

— and no powerful friends in the halls of government...
Civilizations have destroyed themselves by destroying their
farmland. This irremediable loss, never enough noticed, has
been made worse by the huge monocultures and continuous
soil-exposure of the agriculture we now practice.[384]

This system is clearly flawed from an environmental and a nutritional
standpoint. The use of our most important factor in food production — the
soil — is simply unsustainable within the industrial-agricultural model. An
old saying attributed to the Chinese states wisely, "Humankind, despite its
artistic pretensions, its sophistication, and its many accomplishments, owes
its existence to a six-inch layer of topsoil and the fact that it rains."
Preserving the topsoil is in our best interest; building the topsoil is our best
strategy.

Monocrops also divert water from natural habitats. Globally, agriculture
accounts for 80-90% of all freshwater used by humans.[385] The necessity of
irrigation is based on crops planted in areas where they otherwise wouldn't be
able to survive. This bolsters production in those areas, but it also destroys the
natural habitats that rely on those water sources. It's water pulled from lakes,
rivers, and streams, requiring dams and all the celebrated symbols of progress
that dramatically alter the natural landscape and spell death for beavers, trout,
sparrows, and countless other species that call the waters home.

Monocrops have already taken over most of the fertile land available,
wiping out countless ecosystems. Lierre Keith asks the important questions:

I'm not asking, How many people can be fed? but a very different
question: How can people be fed? Not, What feeds the most people?
but What feeds people sustainably? We need a full accounting. The
absolute bottom line is: what methods of food production build

---

[384] Jackson and Berry (2009). "A 50-Year Farm Bill." *New York Times.*

[385] Morison et al (2008). Improving water use in crop production. *Philosophical Transactions of the Royal Society Biological Sciences* 363(1491): 639–658.

topsoil while using only ambient sun and rain? *Because nothing else is sustainable.*[386]

Perhaps the problem is with the conventional understanding of sustainability, which seeks to maximize the human population without furthering the destruction we see all around us. It's a measured approach, starting from where we are now instead of where we can be. Is that even a fair pursuit? Is it a reasonable promise that there will be fewer oil spills in the future? Less habitat eviscerated? Healthier foodstuffs grown in less fertile soil? Is this a safe bet, or blind optimism based on the myth of progress?

And all of this so far is just plant agriculture. Add animals, and the additional harm done by animal food production, under an industrialized system, only further degrades the environment. A Pew Commission report states,

> Industrial Farmed Animal Production systems are largely unregulated, and many practices common to this method of production threaten public health, the environment, animal health and well-being, and rural communities. The use of antibiotics in animals without a diagnosed illness, the mismanagement of the large volumes of farm waste, and the treatment of animals in intensive operations are all of deep concern.[387]

Flaws in animal production methods are relatively well-known, thanks to vocal vegetarians, vegans, and animal rights groups. Farm animals are easy to see. They're in our grocery stores, our plates, and our countryside. But there's far more injustice in what we don't see: the habitats our industrial models

---

[386]Keith, p 126.

[387] Pew Commission (2007). Putting Meat on the Table: Industrial Farmed Animal Production in America. pp. 21. [PDF Web file] Retrieved from https://spark-public.s3.amazonaws.com/foodsys/Pew.PuttingMeatontheTable.2007.v2.pdf

destroy, the rivers now stagnant and putrefied, the species that are gone forever. And it's due to both animal and plant agriculture. This is the truth overlooked by vegetarians with grain-based diets. It's the blind spot in their worldview. We have to accept this truth in order to move past it and find real sustainability.

There is a more strategic option than industrial agriculture, one that is rooted in the logic of the land. It's a strategy that achieves ecological harmony according to the laws of nature, one that proactively benefits the environment and creates ecologies rather than destroys them.

Sustaining a Sustainable Sustainability

True sustainability has the promise to not only stop the destruction of the environment, but also to rejuvenate much of the harm that's already done. A truly sustainable system would not only mimic the mechanisms of nature that contribute to the enduring cycle of life; they would take control and leverage them in order to improve ecologies and maximize net life in a given area. Like Darwin's terraforming project on Ascension island or the diversity of domesticated and friendly canines, the hands of mankind hold the promise to guide nature; in this case, to guide the elements of nature that lead to a self-sustaining system. And in terms of food production, this is something that is already being done.

Joel Salatin is perhaps the most popular voice for exactly this kind of farming. Featured in movies, magazines, books, and newspapers, *The New York Times* calls him the "High Priest of the Pasture" and describes his operation as an "innovative" and "integrated system on a holistic farm":

> Salatin's secret is the grass, and it is in the pasture that everything begins and ends. He believes that every square yard of sward should contain at least 40 varieties of plants, and he calls his fields a "salad bar," a riot of fescues and clovers and earthworms churning the soil. Cattle graze freely on a patch of

this super-rich pasture, held in by an electrified wire. Every day or so, they are moved to a new patch, and a succession of chickens (or turkeys, in season) are moved into the plot that the cows just left. Both laying chickens and broilers -- raised for their meat -- have portable shelters for shade and are protected from predators by portable webbed polyethylene fencing interlaced with electrified wire. Buried, pond-fed plastic pipes channel pressurized water, virtually anywhere, on demand. The chickens dig through fresh cowpatties for nutritious grubs and worms, and then scratch the manure into the dirt, aerating the soil and creating compost, so the cycle of growth can begin all over again. [388]

Salatin is a pioneer of efficient farming, leveraging the lessons of ecology to operate as closely as possible within a closed loop. His methods are proven to be productive while benefiting the natural ecology and maintaining high standards of food quality, what he calls "beyond organic."

The small ecosystems he creates contribute greatly to the environment. *Salatin is actually able to build topsoil and improve the land while producing food.* He allows each layer of the ecology to contribute to other layers of the ecology. These intimate inter-relationships drive the system's success. He even relies on natural rainfall, capturing it in an on-site pond to take advantage of the surplus. What's left is a surprisingly productive, eternally sustainable system that produces high quality food for local people.

There are many other systems like this. Bill Mollison, an Australian naturalist, was observing marsupials in the Tasmanian rainforest in 1959 when he was struck by the genius of nature. He marveled at the natural ecology, how everything was interconnected, rich with life and teeming in biodiversity. So moved, he recorded in his diary, "I believe that we can build ecosystems that function as well as this one does." Soon, permaculture was

---

[388] Purdum, Todd S. "High Priest of the Pasture." *New York Times.* [Web file] Retrieved from http://query.nytimes.com/gst/fullpage.html?res=9D0CE7DF173EF932A35756C0A9639C8B63

born, defined as "a set of tools for designing natural landscapes that are modeled after nature." [389]

Permaculture, a contraction of 'permanent' and 'agriculture', is a form of sustainable farming. Including many homesteaders (home-farmers), the movement is meant to mimic and create small ecosystems that are self-contained. It led to another form called aquaculture, which raises fish and grows plants simultaneously in a closed system. Together these represent ways that the laws of nature can be leveraged for human benefit.

There are hundreds of farms like these across the country that provide food for local families. In fact, small sustainable farms have been on the rise over the last decade, sprouting up near every major urban center and in towns and cities across the globe. To some degree, these farms grant a little perspective on the money, time, and energy that the agro-industrial complex puts into solving crop yield challenges when sustainability is something that many have already achieved simply by understanding the interconnectedness and resilience of nature.

It's true, though, that much of the world is unsuitable for farms like these. People in remote or ecologically challenging locations have come to rely on conventional monocropping in order to support their large numbers, placing importance on the future of crop management, especially as large populations continue to grow. Most small organic farms today are less productive, but some, like Salatin's, produce at rates comparable to grain-producing industrial farms, on a food calorie per acre basis. [390] The difference between the two is that polyculture farming contributes to the environment and monocropping destroys it. Depending on where we live, many of us are fortunate to have the ability to support sustainable farming systems, an important step toward environmental progress.

---

[389] Hemenway, Toby. *Gaia's Garden*. Chelsea Green, 2009. p 5.
[390] Keith, p 101.

Strategies in Sustainability

Support local sustainable farms. Finding the right farm near you will be worth the investment, for your physical and mental health, and for the planet. **Choose ethically raised animals.** These animals get to live out healthy lives, and you're healthier for it, too. **Grow your own food.** Homesteading can be fun for the right personality, and you'll be helping to create more life in the process! **Minimize car use.** Living without a car is inconvenient and, for some, impossible. If you're lucky enough to live somewhere that it's possible, give it a shot. You may find it liberating and morally rewarding. **Rethink how many kids you want to have.** Kahlil Gibran once said, "Your children are not your children. They are the sons and daughters of life's longing for itself." Perhaps the most difficult decision of all, rethinking children means rethinking an entire cultural value system.

Full Circle: a Final Thought

By now we have addressed a great deal. We have explored the roles of science, logic, and strategy in decision-making. We have covered the natural history of the human animal. We have considered the intersections between diet, exercise, sleep, happiness, love, nature, morality, and sustainability. And now I'd like to point out the heavy truth that everything is connected.

Psychologists have long known about the stages of personal development. As we mature, our consciousness, our cares, and our values change dramatically. We go from being relatively self-centered to being relatively selfless. In fact, the loss of selfishness is a defining characteristic of the adult. Adults learn to care for their kids, their grandchildren, their families, their communities, all the while finding meaning and value in those relationships as their conscience opens to others. How far can we go in this direction of human virtue? We're already a couple of degrees away from caring about the planet and everyone in it.

Science has demonstrated that you can't be happy unless you eat right, because your mind and body are connected intimately. We also know that the happiest people in the world are the ones that leverage their evolved psychologies by devoting their lives to a higher purpose, often selfless yet self-actualizing. Relevant to this chapter, choosing healthy food from a sustainable farm creates a closed loop in this interconnected system, ultimately providing meaning and value by fueling the virtue of protecting the planet and also the utility of eating healthy. As a culture, honoring our bodies, loving our kin, forging strong communities, defending our planet, and building a promising future — these are our highest virtues as a species. And no discussion about happiness is relevant without them.

Civilization has unfurled a system of systems that simultaneously adds and detracts from our lives in myriad ways, most of which we have covered. Seeing that fact clearly and exploring its nuances will help us see ourselves and our society for what it is, and will help us see the future for what it can be.

As this book came together, my head was buried in one detail after the next. It wasn't until the end that I looked up and discovered that I had been unearthing pieces of a puzzle. And staring at the pieces, it was an easy puzzle to solve.

When you boil down the psychological facts of happiness, and marry that with the evolutionary perspective on human virtue, you start to see a picture emerging of a transcendent species, one whose evolved architecture leads to behaviors that belie its "lowly origins," as Darwin once remarked. We aren't simply animals fighting to downplay the ugly truths of our nature. We are also animals seeking to overcome our nature, to rise above the inner turmoil that exists between our comprising evolved traits and modern lives.

There is no doubt that there are dark truths eternally embedded into human nature. But their exploration inevitably leads to a positive conclusion: that there is good in us. *The good in us can be leveraged.* And when it is, we are better for it, for we walk the paths of gods.

Everything that transcends the human animal to form the human being is rooted in our evolutionary heritage. Everything that gives the future hope and the world meaning is etched into our bones. We ought to be happy. It's a gift from nature. We ought to be united. It's in our blood. We ought to be good to others, righteous in our own eyes, and virtued as highly as ambition allows. This is the path nature has laid out for us. We must simply choose it. We must act.

"It is perfectly true, as philosophers say, that life must be understood backwards. But they forget the other proposition, that it must be lived forwards."

Soren Kierkegaard

the first existentialist

THE END

APPENDIX A: RESOURCES

Books

Nutrition and Physical Degeneration by Weston A. Price

Disease and Western Civilization by Staffan Lindeberg

The Paleo Diet by Loren Cordain

The Primal Blueprint by Mark Sisson

The Paleo Solution by Robb Wolf

The Human Diet: its Origin and Evolution edited by Peter S. Ungar and Mark F. Teaford

Protein Power by Michael Eades

Primal Body, Primal Mind by Nora Gedgaudas

Lights Out! Sleep, Sugar, and Survival by T.S. Wiley

Perfect Health Diet by Paul Jaminet

Why We Get Fat by Gary Taubes

The New Evolution Diet by Art de Vany

In Defense of Food by Michael Pollan

The Vegetarian Myth by Lierre Keith

Know Your Fats by Mary Enig

Catching Fire by Richard Wrangham

Fat and Cholesterol are Good For You by Uffe Ravnskov

Going Against the Grain by Melissa Diane Smith

Against the Grain by Richard Manning

Deadly Harvest by Geoff Bond

The How of Happiness by Sonja Lyubomirsky

Thinking Strategically by Dixit and Nalebuff

Genome by Matt Ridley

Darwinian Happiness by Bjorn Grinde

Websites

hackingevolution.com
evolvify.com
ancestryfoundation.org
arthurdevany.com
marksdailyapple.com
chriskresser.com
westonaprice.org
robbwolf.com
paleodiet.com

Movies

The Perfect Human Diet (2012)
Science of Dogs (2007)
Dirt! The Movie (2009)
Farmageddon (2011)
Fat Head (2009)
Food Fight (2008)
Food, Inc. (2008)

APPENDIX B: SAMPLE MEAL PLANS, BY COST

For the Starving Musician:

Tips:

- DON'T EAT OUT.
- Cook in quantities to save money on bulk purchases and to have leftovers.
- Keep an eye out for sale items and buy in bulk, freezing what you won't use for later.
- For veggies, stick to the basics, like carrots, cabbage, squash, celery, cauliflower, spinach, kale, etc. All very inexpensive.
- For meat, buy and cook whole birds. Eat lots of eggs, sardines, and organ meats; they're often less than $1 per meal. Buy red meats and fish, if you must, when they are on sale.
- For carbs, include white rice and peeled potatoes in the diet in addition to carbs like sweet potatoes and cassava when possible.

*Prices are slightly overestimated to 2013 numbers to provide a buffer, and are based on what I normally see in California markets. Also based on big portions, so expect to spend less if your appetite is smaller.

Breakfast: Veggie scramble, plus fruit — $2.10

3 eggs — $0.60 ¼ onion — $0.15 ½ tomato — $0.40 ½ bell pepper — $0.50 olive oil and butter — $0.20 banana — $0.25	Pan fry onions and bell pepper in olive oil and butter combo on medium for 3 minutes. Add tomato for 1 min. Crack in 3 eggs and stir occasionally until ready. Have a banana for dessert!

Lunch/Dinner:: Tuna-Veggie stir-fry — $3.60

4-6 spears asparagus — $1 ½ onion — $0.30 1 can tuna — $1 1 can water chestnuts — $1 1 cup white rice — $0.10 soy sauce cumin salt and pepper 1 tsp sesame oil — $0.20	Start rice in rice cooker or pot. Pan fry onion and asparagus in butter on medium for 5 minutes. Add shoots and chestnuts, soy sauce, tuna, sesame oil, and spices. Stir and leave 1 minute, then serve over rice. Add soy sauce to taste.

Lunch/Dinner: Taco salad — $2.90

¼ lb ground turkey — $1 ¼ onion — $0.15 ¼ cup cooked black beans — $0.25 2 oz shredded cheddar cheese — $0.30 1 head romaine lettuce — $1 2 tbsp sour cream — $0.20	Pan fry turkey, beans, and onion in olive oil until cooked thoroughly. Serve over bed of chopped lettuce. Top with sour cream and cheddar.

For the Average Joe

Tips:

- Stick to pastured animal products when possible.

Breakfast: Bacon and eggs, plus fruit — $2.50

2 strips pastured bacon — $1.00 3 omega-3 eggs — $0.70 ¼ avocado — $0.30 ¼ cantaloupe — $0.50	Pan fry bacon until desired crispness. Pour out fat, leaving the residue for flavor. Add eggs, turn as desired. Top with avocado and follow with cantaloupe.

Lunch: Chicken lettuce wraps — $2.90

1 chicken breast — $2 butter 3 sheets romaine — $0.50 ¼ avocado — $0.30 salt and pepper parmesan — $0.10	Pan fry chicken breast in butter, then chop into small pieces. Add to inside of each romaine sheet and top with salt, pepper, avocado, and parmesan.

Dinner: Corned beef, cabbage, and beer — $5.75 per meal

4 lb corned beef brisket — $18 1 head of white cabbage — $2 1 gluten-free sorghum beer or hard cider — $1.25	This is simple and yields tons of leftovers. Simmer brisket in pot of water for three hours until tender and flaky. Quarter the cabbage and add to soup for 15 minutes. Remove from broth or serve as soup. Pair with sorghum beer or cider.

For the Optimal Eater

Tips:

○ Always choose pastured animal products. Prefer wild-caught fish and grass-finished ruminants (wagyu beef, lamb, bison, deer, elk) over pork and poultry.

○ Check out as many local farms as possible in order to find the one that suits you best (organic, permaculture, and biodynamic farms are a great choice).

○ Include fermented foods in the diet such as sauerkraut, kimchi, and kombucha.

○ Consider joining a CSA (Community-Supported Agriculture). They ship you a box full of fresh fruits and vegetables for a reasonable fee, straight to your door.

○ Never cook higher than medium heat. 'Low and slow' is the way to go.

○ Avoid burning foods while cooking.

○ Add broth to as many meals as possible. In addition to soups and stews, add broth to stir-frys, mashed potatoes, omelets, whatever you can!

○ Supplement with Vitamin K2, D3, probiotics, magnesium, fish or krill oil, and a multivitamin.

*Prices not included because they should be irrelevant to the truly optimal eater. You don't need to be rich to eat this way, though. It's still cheaper than eating at restaurants.

Lunch: Chicken-potato-leek soup

2 chicken breasts 3 quarts free-range chicken broth 1 leek ½ onion 2 cloves garlic 3 acorn squash 2 large golden potatoes 4 tbsp olive oil butter rosemary sage thyme salt and Pepper	Great for leftovers. Bring large pot of 3 quarts broth to boil then reduce to simmer. Skin potatoes, chop and add to broth. Add chopped leek, onion, minced garlic, and chopped squash. Simmer for 10 minutes. Pan fry chicken breast in butter on medium until golden, then chop into bite-size squares and add to soup along with spices and olive oil. Stir and simmer 3-5 minutes, allow to cool, then serve.

Dinner: Steak and potatoes

½ lb grass-finished steak 1 organic sweet potato 1 organic italian squash (zucchini) pastured butter salt and pepper 1 glass red wine	Bring the steak to room temperature and coat with melted butter and salt. Place on the grill at medium heat for 3-6 minutes per side. Quarter the italian squash lengthwise and pan fry on medium in olive oil, salt, and pepper. Slice sweet potato into ½ inch pieces and boil for 10-15 minutes until soft. Pair with red wine.

Lunch/Dinner: Apple-baked tenderloin and spinach salad

2-3 lb pork tenderloin 2 tbsp butter 2 cups apple cider 1 cinnamon stick 4 cloves 1 pinch nutmeg 4-6 cups raw spinach ¼ cup dried organic cranberries walnuts 3 oz goat cheese 4 tbsp olive oil 1 tbsp balsamic vinegar 1 shallot	Set oven to 350 degrees. Coat tenderloin in salt and melted butter, place in over for 30 minutes. In small pot, add two cups spiced apple cider, cinnamon, cloves, nutmeg, butter, and heat on low and stir for 5 minutes. Baste spiced apple cider onto top and sides of tenderloin every 5 minutes until done. Turn the tenderloin once halfway through. In a large bowl, place spinach, cranberries, walnuts, goat cheese, diced shallot. Top with olive oil and balsamic. Feeds four people, or great for leftovers.

SPECIAL THANKS

Mom and Pop, Guchi, Lila, and Ron, Bobo and Lala, my family, thank you for your love and support throughout three chaotic years of obsessive writing and researching. To my circles of friends, thank you for helping me to understand tribe, to know firsthand the depths of what I'm writing about. To my teachers and mentors, all of them, thank you for however slightly guiding me to this place in life, preparing me for what I see as some of the most important work of our time. To all those before me who helped to build this beautiful tapestry of human knowledge, thank you for the honor and glory of being the next one to help.

Lydia Johnson, you made this book possible by being my everything during the most revolutionary period of my life, a time of tremendous change, learning, and self-discovery. Thank you so much. Jen Cameron, my intrepid companion, you have helped me in ways unimaginable by exploring with me the depths of the human heart and soul. Colin Triplett and Andreas Herczeg, thank you for making this book better. Thank you. Thank you all.

INDEX